# Dental Extractions Made Easier

### Brook A. Niemiec, DVM

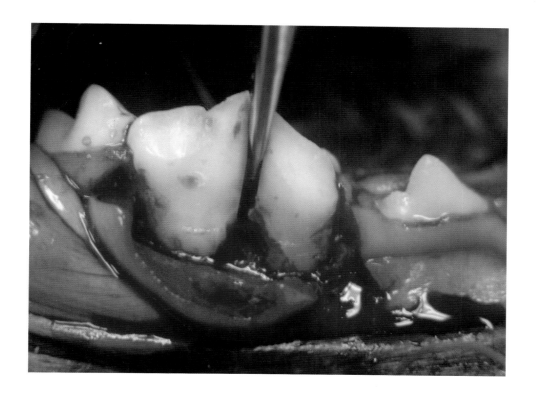

## Practical Veterinary Publishing
5775 Chesapeake Court
San Diego, CA 92123
USA

# Additional publications by the author include:

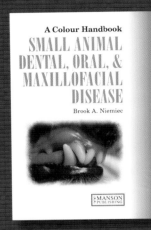

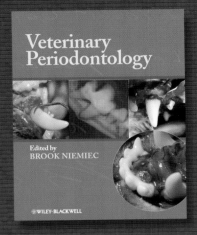

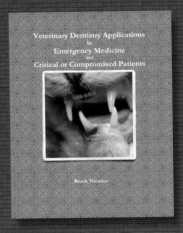

**Oral Diseases Color Handbook:** A quick reference guide to oral diseases in the dog and cat.

**Veterinary Periodontology:** The definitive text for veterinary periodontology. This book covers the subject from basic to advanced with full color step-by-step procedures. Numerous new techniques and research throughout.

**Emergency Veterinary Dentistry:** A reference guide for veterinary emergency care as well as a guide for proper therapy of critical and compromised patients.

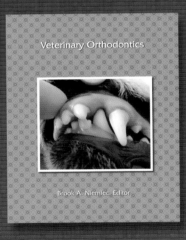

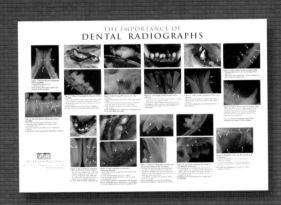

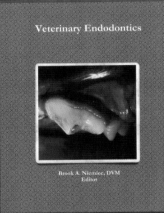

**Veterinary Orthodontics:** The first book dedicated wholly to veterinary orthodontics. Lean how to tackle this common problem with expert guidance.

**Client Educational Poster:** A picture is worth 1000 words! Use this poster to inform your clients about the importance of dental radiology. **An 8 ½ X 11 "Drawer sized" poster is also available.**

**Veterinary Endodontics:** The first book dedicated wholly to veterinary endodontics. Includes chapters on restoration, surgical endodontics, and avoiding & fixing common errors.

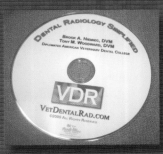

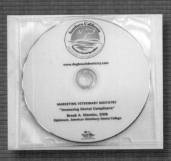

**Dental Radiology Simplified Video:** Let our team of experts guide you and your staff through proper positioning techniques, digital radiology techniques, and avoiding common errors.

**Marketing Veterinary Dentistry Video:** In this live recording, Dr. Niemiec combines exhaustive research with years of experience communicating with clients in both general and specialty practice to give you the information to make the most out of your dental department.

For ordering information please visit  www.practicalvetpublishing.com

# Table of Contents

Copyright 2012, Practical Veterinary Publishing

Practical Veterinary Publishing
5775 Chesapeake Court, San Diego, CA
United States of America
**ISBN: 978-0-9852148-2-1**

**Introduction:**

Dental extractions are a very common surgical procedure, typically performed daily in most veterinary practices, yet they are **not** a simple undertaking. As such, they should be approached with the same level of preparation as any other surgical procedure.

Regardless of tooth size, all single root extractions should start with the 10 steps as outlined below. Multi-root teeth require sectioning into single rooted pieces, which are then treated as single root extractions. Finally, large teeth or any difficult/complicated presentations (due to root malformations), are best extracted following the creation of gingival flaps and removal of bone.

Dental extractions are typically performed to remove infected and/or painful teeth. Indications include, but are not limited to: endodontic disease (i.e. fractured or intrinsically stained teeth), severe periodontal disease, traumatic malocclusion, persistent or infected deciduous teeth, tooth resorption, abscessed teeth, caudal stomatitis, and unerupted teeth.[1, 2] It must be noted however, that options such as root canal therapy or periodontal surgery can effectively save many of these teeth and therefore should be offered **prior** to considering extraction.[1] In fact, in this author's experience, abscessed teeth without concurrent root resorption carry a good prognosis with root canal therapy.

Complete extraction of the diseased tooth almost invariably resolves the existing disease state (pain and/or infection). However, if extractions are improperly performed, even simple procedures can have numerous iatrogenic complications including: hemorrhage, osteomyelitis, oronasal fistula, forcing of a root tip into the mandibular canal or nasal cavity, jaw fracture, ocular damage, etc.[1,3-5] The most common iatrogenic complication (by far) is leaving retained tooth roots behind.[1, 6, 7] This generally results in continued infection in and around the retained root.[2,6 ,7] It is exceedingly unusual for animal patients to show overt clinical signs, but they suffer regardless. Occasionally, this problem causes a draining tract from the retained roots, which could result in a malpractice claim.[1]

A guideline for proper and successful dental extractions is summarized in the following 10 steps. These steps constitute the technique for a single rooted tooth, but also for multirooted teeth which are treated the same way following sectioning, and for large teeth following bone removal. **This book is an excellent guide for extraction procedures, but skills are best learned via hands on wetlabs. For a list of wetlabs taught by the author please visit www.dogbeachvet.com.**

## Step 1: **OBTAIN CONSENT**

Never extract a tooth without prior owner consent, no matter how advanced the problem is, or how obvious it may be that extraction is the proper therapy.[1,8,9] Consent should preferably be written, but is acceptable verbally via a phone call. Be sure to have a (or several) valid daytime numbers for the client and inform them they must be available during surgery hours. Another very effective means to contact clients is to check out/loan pagers to them for the day.

If the client cannot be reached and prior consent was not obtained, do **not** pull the tooth.[9] Document the problem, recover the patient and reschedule the work. Remember, the tooth can always be extracted later, but it cannot be put back in.

## Step 2: <u>EXPOSE PRE-OPERATIVE DENTAL RADIOGRAPHS</u>

Dental radiographs should be made of all teeth prior to commencing the extraction.[1,5,10] Dental radiographs are invaluable resources for guiding the practitioner through the extraction process. Radiographs allow the practitioner to determine the amount of disease present, any root abnormalities (Figures 1 and 2), or resorption/ankylosis (Figure 3).[1,5,10] (Note: approximately 10% of feline maxillary third premolars have a third root.)[11] Significant mandibular alveolar bone loss secondary to periodontal disease weakens the bone, and predisposes patients to an iatrogenic pathologic fracture (Figure 4).[12] This is most common with the canine and first molar teeth in small and toy breed dogs, due to the proportionally larger size of the tooth roots of these teeth compared to the jaw.[13] Dentoalveolar ankylosis makes extraction by traditional elevation practically impossible. For this reason, crown amputation and intentional root retention is acceptable for advanced Type 2 feline tooth resorption, but it is important to make this distinction prior to treatment decisions.[14] (see pages 44-46 for a complete discussion of the indications and techniques for crown amputation). In summary, dental radiographs provide critical information for treatment planning and the successful outcome of dental extraction procedures. In addition, radiographs provide solid evidence in the medical record.[10]

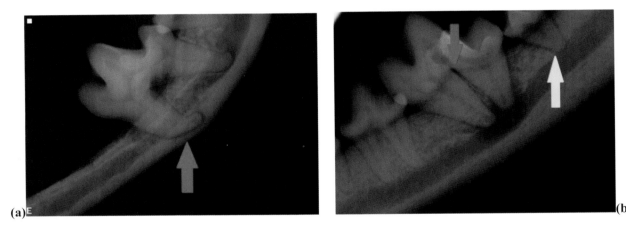

(a)

(b)

**Figure 1: Malformed roots of "normal appearing" teeth.**
**Variations which would greatly complicate the extraction procedure**
  a) **Mandibular first molar of a toy breed dog with a curved mesial root. (red arrow)**
     **Note also, the apex is very close to the ventral cortex.**
  b) **Mandibular first and second molar of a small breed dog. The first molar (309) has invergent roots (red arrow), which would complicate sectioning. This tooth also has periapical rarefaction. The second molar (310) (which normally has two roots) is single rooted. (blue arrow)**

2

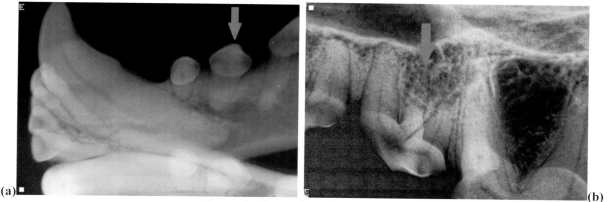

Figure 2: Unusual number of roots.
This is critical knowledge when sectioning teeth for extraction.
a)   Mandibular second premolar (in a dog) with only one root. (red arrow)
b)   Maxillary third premolar (in a dog) with three roots. (red arrow points at palatine root)

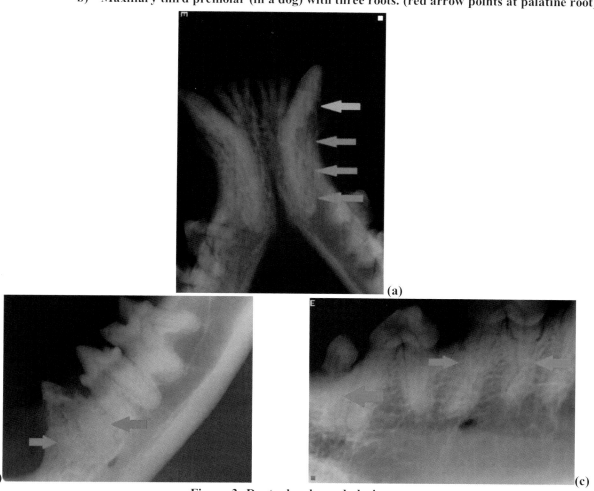

Figure 3: Dentoalveolar ankylosis.
a) The mandibular canines in a cat. b) Mandibular third premolar in a cat.
c) Demonstrates a similar process in the mandibular premolars of a dog.
The resorption is shown by the red arrows.  The blue arrow in figure 3a shows the small clinical lesion in this case.  Note, the clinical lesion is minimal, but the root involvement is significant.
The third premolar in figure (b) and the first premolar in figure (c) are candidates for crown amputation.

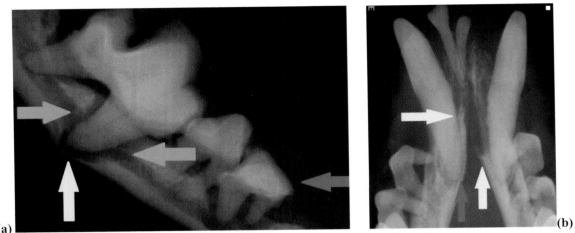

(a)                                                                                                    (b)

Figure 4: Severe alveolar bone loss in the mandible of small/toy breed dogs.
These images reveal areas of significant alveolar bone loss in the area of the mandibular first molar (a) and canines (b) resulting in minimal remaining bone surrounding the roots (yellow arrows).
The blue arrows in image (a) show the vertical bone loss; while the red arrow shows the third premolar which has lost all attachment and is held in the jaw by a "calculus bridge".
Note, the yellow arrow in figure (a) and the red arrow in figure (b) reveal the very minimal amount of bone apical to the tooth roots, even without periodontal disease present.
This is critical information in order to avoid iatrogenic jaw fracture during the extraction procedure.

## Step 3: <u>OBTAIN PROPER VISABILITY AND ACCESSIBILITY</u>[1,9]

Patients should be positioned to allow maximum visibility of the surgical area and for the surgeon to be most comfortable and therefore more successful. This author finds dorsal recumbency to be best for most extractions, except in the case of the mandibular premolar and molars where lateral recumbancy (with the affected side up) provides superior access. Ideal patient positioning may change during the extraction procedure and adjustments should be made as needed. Surgical lighting is best when bright and focused on the surgical field. Suction, air/water syringes, and gauze should be utilized continually to keep the surgical field clear, and appropriate (non-traumatic) mouth gags can be used to hold the mouth in open position. Even proper mouth gags should be removed occasionally to allow relaxation of the joint and decrease post-op discomfort. Finally, magnification can be useful to locate furcations or retained root tips. Many dentists use head loupes which combine magnification and lighting.[a]

---

[a] Perioptix, Carlsbad, CA

4

# Step 4: **PAIN MANAGEMENT**

Extractions are surgical procedures which are moderately to severely painful. A multimodal approach typically provides superior analgesia and safety.[15-18]

Opioids are excellent pain medications and are safe for virtually all patients, including those with metabolic complications (renal and hepatic disease). Morphine, hydromorphone, and buprenorphine are good options. Fentanyl patches may provide long lasting pain control without oral administration. Butorphanol is **not** adequate for pain control as it provides limited pain relief for only approximately 23-53 minutes.[19]

Non-steroidal anti-inflammatories (NSAIDs) are an excellent means of providing pain control for oral surgery, with the advantage of (typically) 24 hours of efficacy. In fact, a pre-op NSAID injection can be especially advantageous for the initial post-operative period when the patient may be anorectic and not taking oral meds. NSAIDs should be used with caution in feline patients and in cases of metabolic disease, especially renal impairment. Pre-operative testing (including urinalysis) and close intraoperative blood pressure monitoring is critical to minimize anesthetic complications.

Reports indicate that acute surgical pain applied to chronically diseased/painful tissue actually heightens the pain response, making it more difficult to manage post-operatively. Preemptive analgesia is proven to be more effective than post-operative, making it important to administer the drugs **before** the painful procedure.[15-18, 20]

For lengthy or complicated procedures, other systemic medications can be considered such as lidocaine, micro doses of dissociatives (ketamine or alpha 2 agonists), and CRIs of fentanyl. The reader is directed to an anesthesia/analgesia text for further review of these techniques. An additional, yet critical, method of pain management is regional anesthesia, also known as local nerve blocks. When properly performed, regional anesthesia provides complete local analgesia, which markedly decreases MAC and improves recovery.

The two agents commonly used for regional anesthesia are lidocaine and bupivacaine. Lidocaine has a fast onset of 1-2 minutes, but a relatively short duration, lasting only 1-2 hours.[18, 21] It therefore does not provide adequate analgesic duration for lengthy procedures. Furthermore, lidocaine offers minimal if any pain relief in the postoperative period. Conversely, bupivacaine's analgesic effect is significantly longer in duration, lasting 6-8 hours.[18, 21] Concerns with its use were based on a longer onset of action, but human studies reveal it may take effect in as little as 4.4 to 7.7 minutes.[22-24] Maximizing the benefits of short onset with longer duration made combining these products a popular option.[25,26] However, recent research has shown that combining lidocaine and bupivacaine may result in decreased efficacy.[27] Local anesthetic agents are vasodilative, and thus stimulate faster drug removal and a shorter duration of action. The addition of epinephrine to local agents can increase the activity by 50%.[28] Furthermore, adding either buprenorphine or morphine to bupivacaine may result in a duration of effect almost twice that of bupivacaine alone.[29] This author utilizes plain bupivacaine exclusively, as 6-8 hours is sufficient efficacy for patient comfort, without lasting too long into the post-operative period to potentially compromise eating.

While there is some concern with marcaine use and cardiotoxicity in cats, avoiding intravenous injection and overdosage will eliminate this complication. For this reason, it is critical to aspirate prior to each injection of local anesthetic.[18] If blood is encountered, the needle should be redirected (and reaspirated) to insure that intravenous (or intra-arterial) injection is not performed. When injecting the anesthetic solution, it is best to place a finger gently over the foramen to keep it within the foramen and improve diffusion.

Recommended infusion volumes vary from 0.1ml – 1.6 ml for small to large size patients.[30] The published maximum recommended total dose of local anesthetics is 2 mg/kg (single agent or combination).[18] This level is easy to reach in small patients when utilizing 2% lidocaine. For example, a 5 kg patient should receive a maximum dose of 0.5 cc of 2% lidocaine. Consequently, it is advised to dilute this product to decrease the possibility of overdosage. These guidelines are being reviewed, as the published maximum dose is based on intravenous injection and some anesthesiologists are utilizing much higher dosage for local injections.

The three major nerve blocks used for dental surgery are the infraorbital, mental, and mandibular blocks. Some dentists/anesthesiologists utilize the caudal maxillary block, but this author does not recommend it due to the risk of orbital penetration. If properly performed, the infraorbital block can effectively anesthetize the entire ipsilateral maxillary quadrant.[31]

The depth to which the needle is placed within the foramen is one of significant debate. For the infraorbital block, some dentists recommend that the foramen be just barely or not entered, while others place the needle very deep within the canal to block the molar teeth. This author compromises to somewhere in between (see individual blocks below). Finally, when placing intraforamenal blocks (especially the mental), some authors recommend placing the needle just barely within the foramen to avoid damage to the nerve.

**Infraorbital block:** (Figure 5)

The infraorbital block is effective for the ipsilateral maxilla, teeth, and associated soft tissues. The infraorbital canal runs rostrally just above the apices of the maxillary fourth premolar and exits the maxilla over the distal root of the third premolar. To approximate the dorso-ventral location, it is helpful to imagine the fourth premolar as being approximately the same size mesio-distal as corono-apical. Therefore, first measure the width of the tooth and then also that same distance dorsally from the cusp tip. The infraorbital canal is just apical to this point. The foramen is easily palpated, especially in cats and large breed dogs.

Manually retract the lip and infraorbital neurovascular bundle dorsally. The neurovascular bundle is easily palpated as a band of tissue coursing rostral and slightly dorsal from the infraorbital foramen demonstrated beneath the vestibular mucosa. Advance the needle in a caudal direction, close to the maxillary bone and ventral to the retracted bundle, to a point just inside the canal. The needle should pass into the canal without engaging bone. Correct placement can be confirmed by gentle lateral movement of the needle, allowing it to engage the canal wall. In cats, the infraorbital canal is VERY short, and this may easily allow for orbital penetration.[18] For this reason, barely enter the foramen and direct the needle ventrally. In dogs, do not advance past the medial canthus of the eye.[18] The medicant and its effect will diffuse distally to the molars if a finger is placed over the foramen for 30-60 seconds after injection.[18]

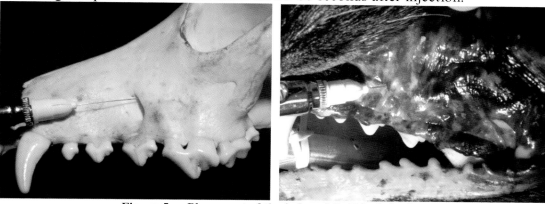

**Figure 5 a: Placement of the infraorbital block in dog.**
**Skull (left) and clinical patient (right).**

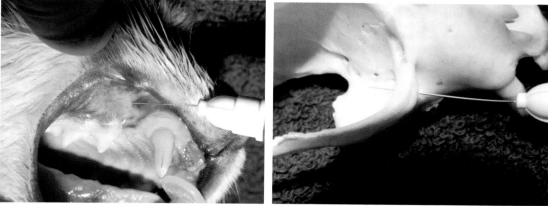

**Figure 5 b: Placement of the infraorbital block in cat.**
**The image on the right demonstrates the short infraorbital canal in a cat.**
**Advance only a short distance into the canal and angle the needle ventrally to avoid orbital penetration.**

**Mental Block:** (Figure 6)

The middle mental foramen is located apical to the mesial root of the second premolar in the dog, at midway in the diastema between the canine tooth and third premolar in the cat,[18, 31] and then approximately 2/3 of the distance ventrally down from the dorsal border of the mandible. Properly performing the mental block affects the inferior alveolar nerve anesthetizing the ipsilateral mandibular first premolar to the central incisor, including the surrounding bone and associated soft tissue.[18, 31] Needle placement must be slightly within the canal to effectively anesthetize all tissue.

To perform this nerve block, the mandibular labial frenulum is retracted ventrally and the needle then inserted at the rostral aspect of the frenulum and advanced at approximately a 45 degree angle along the mandibular bone until it just enters the canal. Placement can be confirmed by moving the syringe laterally to encounter the lateral aspect of the canal.

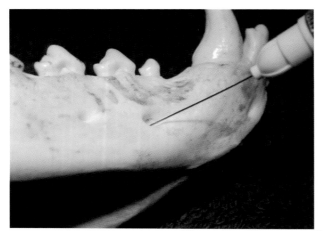 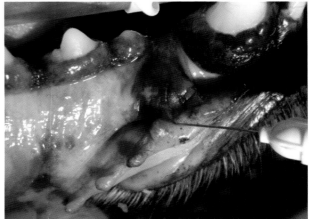

**Figure 6 a: Placement of the mental block in dog.**
**Skull (left) and clinical patient (right).**

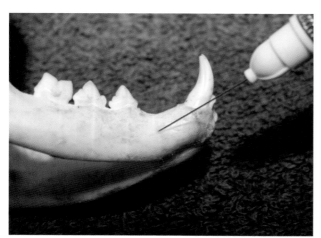 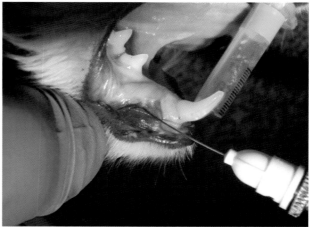

**Figure 6 b: Placement of the mental block in cat.**
**Skull (left) and clinical patient (right).**
**Note the small size of the foramen in the cat.**
**This 27 gauge needle barely fits in the foramen, making this a challenging block in cats and small breed dogs.**

8

**Mandibular Block:** (Figure 7)

The inferior alveolar nerve enters the mandibular foramen on the lingual aspect of the caudal mandible.[31] The caudal mandibular block is performed by infiltrating the nerve at this level prior to its entry into the canal. This block can be performed via either an intra or extra-oral approach, but this author tends to choose the intraoral approach. To perform this method, the patient is placed in dorsal recumbancy with the mouth open. The index finger of the non-dominant hand is used to feel the notch on the ventral aspect of the caudal mandible, and then slid a bit dorsally on the lingual aspect. Using the width measurement of the third molar, the mucosa is entered on the lingual aspect of the mandible, at a point measuring the width of the third molar back from (or distal to) M3. Insert the needle at a 45 degree angle advancing along the bone until the needle is felt moving through the tissues, and inject at this point. If correctly performed, all mandibular teeth, bone, and soft tissue on the treated side are affected by this block.[18]

Patients who are not monitored postoperatively can cause severe trauma to their tongue during the recovery period, but this is extremely rare. Whether these incidents are specifically associated with regional anesthesia or recovery from any procedure is not reflected in the literature. This author has seen it only twice in the past 15 years (both patients were boxers, and one did not have any blocks performed). In any case, proper patient monitoring during recovery should avoid this problem.

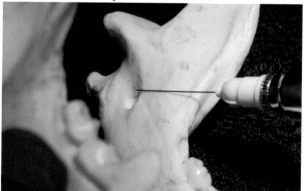 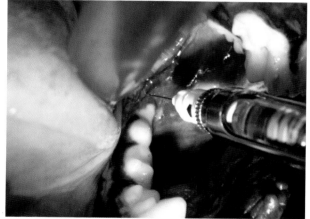

**Figure 7 a: Placement of the mandibular block in dog. Skull (left) and clinical patient (right).**

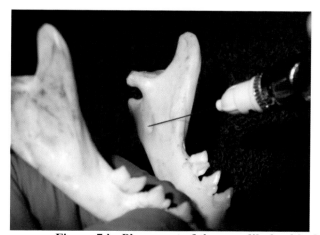 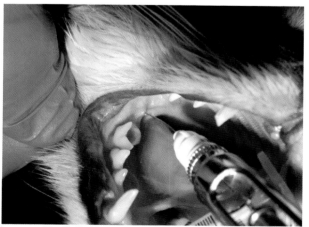

**Figure 7 b: Placement of the mandibular block in cat. Skull (left) and clinical patient (right).**

## Step 5: <u>CUT THE GINGIVAL ATTACHMENT</u> [1,2,7-9,32]

The gingival attachment can be cut with a scalpel blade (number 11 or 15), elevator, or luxator. (Figure 8) The selected instrument is placed into the gingival sulcus with the tip of the blade angled toward the tooth. (a) This helps to avoid cutting along the bone and creating a mucosal defect, or cutting through the gingiva. The blade is then advanced apically to the level of the alveolar bone (b), and carefully continued around the entire tooth circumference.

This step is very helpful in performing extractions as the gingival attachment contributes approximately15% of the retentive strength of the periodontal apparatus. More importantly however, this step will keep the gingiva from tearing during the extraction procedure. It is especially useful with mobile teeth where little elevation is needed, but one edge is still attached. Gingival tearing can create defects that require closure or make a planned closure more difficult.

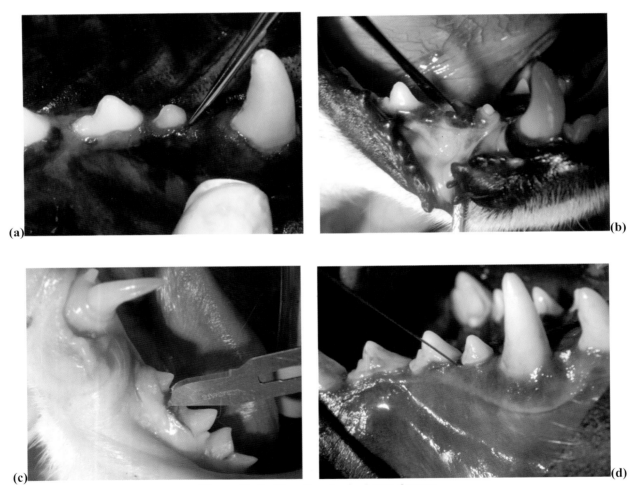

(a)  (b)  (c)  (d)

**Figure 8: Cutting the gingival attachment.**
**Using a luxating elevator (a), a periosteal elevator (b), scalpel blade in a cat (c), and scalpel blade in a dog (d). Note, in all cases the instrument is angled toward the tooth to avoid slipping and potential gingival laceration. In the bottom left (cat) image, note the scalpel blade is too large for this procedure.**

## Step 6: <u>**ELEVATION**</u>

Elevation is the most dangerous step in the extraction procedure. Elevators are sharp surgical instruments which are used in an area of numerous critical and delicate structures. There have been many reports of eyes that have been gouged and lost by extraction instruments as well as at least one confirmed fatality due to an elevator puncturing a patient's brain.[33] In order to avoid causing iatrogenic trauma in the event of instrument slippage or upon encountering diseased bone, the index finger is placed near the tip of the instrument.[2,3,5,9] (Figure 9) In addition, the jaw should be held gently with the opposite hand to provide stability and avoid mandibular fracture.[2]

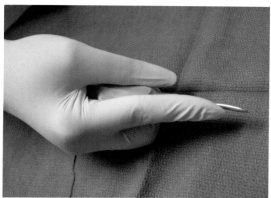

**Figure 9: The instrument is well seated in the palm, with the index finger approximately 1 cm from the tip.**

It is important to select an instrument which matches the curvature and size of the root.[6] In general "go small", as this will result in less pressure and damage. Elevators larger than 3-mm are rarely indicated; generally sizes 1-2 mm work well for cats and 2-3 mm for dogs.

There are numerous instruments available, including the classic elevator as well as luxating and winged types. Classic elevators and winged elevators are used in an "insert and twist" motion to tear the periodontal ligament, whereas luxators are used in a rocking motion during insertion to fatigue as well as cut the periodontal ligament. Luxators may be **gently** twisted for elevation, but they are not designed for this and can be easily damaged when used in this manner.

Elevation is initiated by inserting the instrument firmly yet gently into the periodontal ligament space (between the tooth and the alveolar bone).[2] The insertion should be performed while keeping the instrument at a 10 - 20 degree angle toward the tooth, to avoid slippage.[3] (Figure 10)

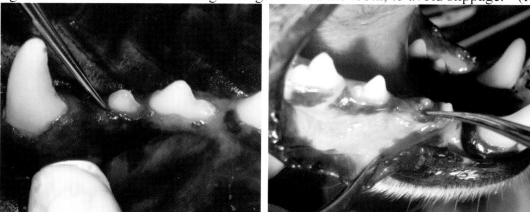

**Figure 10: Elevation.**
**The elevator is placed gently but firmly into the periodontal ligament space.**
**On the right, note how the instrument is angled toward the tooth to avoid slipping.**

Once in the space between the bone and the tooth, the instrument is *gently* twisted with two-finger pressure.[2] (Figure 11) This is not to say that the instrument should be held with two fingers, rather the entire hand (see above) should be used to hold the instrument. Twist only with the force that you could generate when holding with two fingers. Hold the position for 10-30 seconds to fatigue and tear the periodontal ligament.[1,3,6] The tooth should move at least slightly during elevation. If the tooth does not move, no damage is being done to the periodontal ligament.

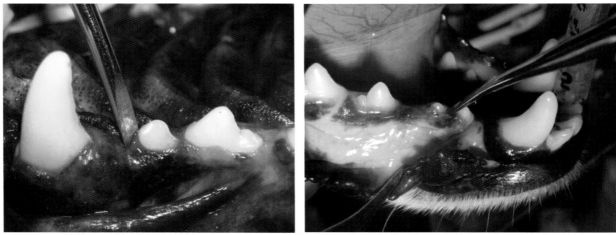

**Figure 11: Once within the periodontal ligament space, the elevator is *gently* twisted.**

The periodontal ligament is very effective in resisting short, intense forces.[34] It is only by the exertion of prolonged force (i.e. 10-30 seconds) that the ligament will become weakened. Increased pressure will transfer much of the force to the alveolar bone and tooth which can result in the fracture of one of these structures. Therefore, it is important to moderate the force. After holding for 10 - 30 seconds, reposition the instrument approximately 1/8 of the way around the tooth and repeat the above step.[1] (Figure 12) Continue this procedure 360 degrees around the tooth, each time moving the elevator apically as much as possible. (Figure 13) Depending on the level of disease and the size of the tooth, a few to several rotations of the tooth may be necessary.

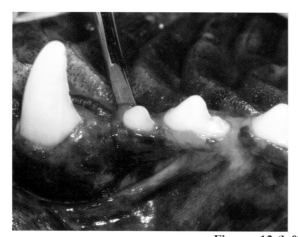 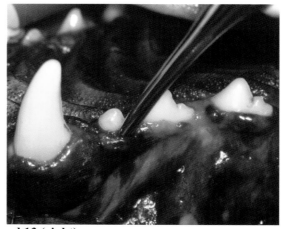

**Figures 12 (left) and 13 (right)**
**Fig 12: After initial elevation, the elevator is replaced approximately 1/8 of the way around the tooth.**
**Fig 13: This continues circumferentially around the tooth, advancing apically.**

Other techniques of elevation utilize the elevator as a wheel and axel.[1] To perform it in this fashion, place the instrument perpendicularly under a ridge of tooth that is at (approximately) the level of the alveolar bone and gently twist.[5,8] (Figure 14) If a natural ledge is not present, one can be created with a dental bur.[35]

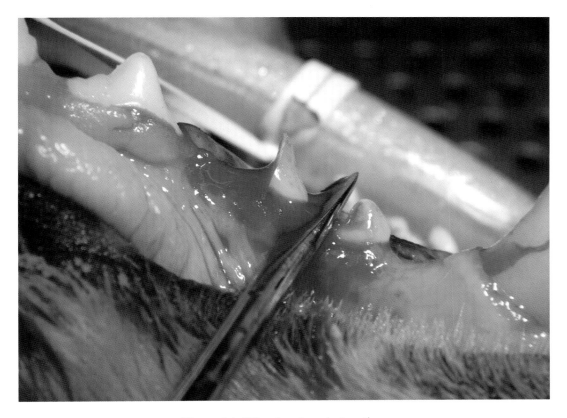

**Figure 14: Wheel and axel elevation.**
**The elevator is positioned perpendicular to the long axis of the tooth,**
**with the edge under the ledge at the cemento-enamel junction (CEG).**
**If a natural ledge is not present, one can be created with a dental bur.**
**Be careful not to involve/damage neighboring teeth.**

The key to successful elevation is PATIENCE.[5,9] Only by slow, consistent elevation will the root loosen without breaking. It is always easier to extract an intact root than to remove fractured root tips.[6]

If elevation is not resulting in tooth mobility in a fairly short period of time, there is a problem. This may be due to faulty extraction technique, or more likely an area of dentoalveolar ankylosis. Review your technique and make sure the elevator is between the tooth and the bone. If technique is correct, review the dental radiographs for signs of ankylosis. If ankylosis is present, a surgical approach should be employed (see below). Dental radiographs are a two dimensional image of a three dimensional space, so small areas of ankylosis may not be radiographically evident. Moreover, if the extraction is not going well, a surgical approach is always an option.

## Step 7: **EXTRACT THE TOOTH**

Removing the tooth should only be attempted after the tooth is very mobile and loose.[2,3] Removal is accomplished by grasping the tooth with the extraction forceps and gently pulling the tooth from the socket.[2,9] (Figure 15) Do NOT apply undue pressure as this may result in root fracture.[2] In many cases, especially with premolars, the roots are round in shape and will respond favorably to *gentle* twisting and holding of the tooth while applying traction.[1, 3, 35] This should not be performed if there are root abnormalities (significant curves, weakening) seen on the pre-operative radiograph.

It is helpful to think of the extraction forceps as an extension of your fingers. Undue pressure should not be applied. If the tooth does not come out easily, more elevation is necessary. Start elevation again until the tooth is loose enough to be easily removed from the alveolus. This is an important point, because root fractures occur more commonly when using extraction forceps than while using elevators. When extraction forceps are applied, not only can the tooth be significantly torqued, but the tooth is typically grasped high on the crown. This action creates a lever, resulting in increased force at the tooth bone interface. In contrast, when an elevator is properly used, the elevator is confined in a tight space, which somewhat limits the amount of force that can be applied.

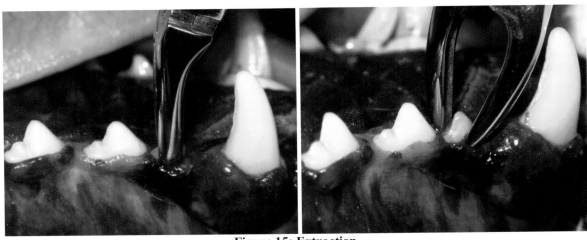

**Figure 15: Extraction.**
**The loosened tooth is carefully grasped with the extraction forceps and removed from the socket.**
**A gentle twist (and hold) is acceptable in many cases (right).**

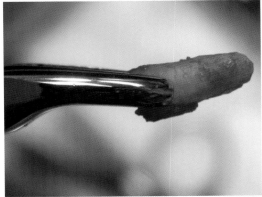

**The extracted tooth: The smooth/round apex is an indication of complete extraction.**
**However, dental radiographs should be exposed regardless of physical appearance. (See below)**

## Step 8: **DEBRIDEMENT & ALVEOLOPLASTY**

This step is performed to remove diseased tissue or bone, or any rough bony edges that could irritate the gingiva and delay healing.[1,5,7,36] Diseased tissue can be removed by hand with a curette. (Figure 16) Bone removal and smoothing is best performed with a coarse diamond bur on a water-cooled high-speed air driven hand-piece.[1,3,5,35,36] (Figure 17) Next, the alveolus should be gently flushed with a 0.12% chlorhexidine solution to decrease bacterial contamination.[5,7,35-38] (Figure 18) After the alveolus is cleaned, it may be packed with an osseopromotive substance[b c.5,37,38] This is done to support the alveolus during healing, provide hemostasis, and help maintain the alveolar ridge.[1,39]

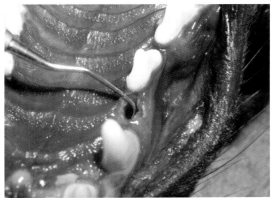

Figure 16: Debriding with a dental curette.

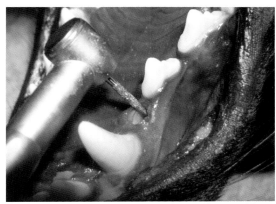

Figure 17: Smoothing bone with a diamond bur.

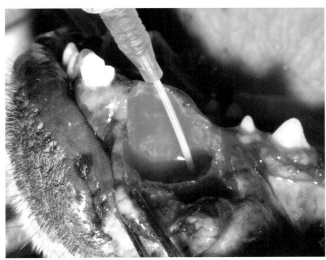

Figure 18: Lavage of the sulcus with a blunt tipped cannula (in this case an IV catheter).

---

[b] Periomix: Veterinary Transplant Services.
[c] Consil: Nutrimax.

## Step 9: <u>**CLOSURE OF THE EXTRACTION SITE**</u>

This is a controversial subject amongst veterinary dentists, and thus some texts recommend closure of only large extractions.[1] However, many authors (including this one) recommend suturing almost all extraction sites. Closure of the extraction site promotes hemostasis and improves post-operative comfort and aesthetics.[3] It is always indicated in cases of larger teeth, or any time that a gingival flap is utilized.[1,35] This is best accomplished with size 3/0 to 5/0 absorbable sutures (e.g chromic gut, vicryl, or monocryl) on a reverse cutting needle.[1,2,36,38] Closure is performed with a simple interrupted pattern, placed 2 to 3-mm apart.[1 5,7 35 36,38] (Figure 19) It is best to utilize one additional throw over manufacturer's recommendations in order to counteract tongue action.

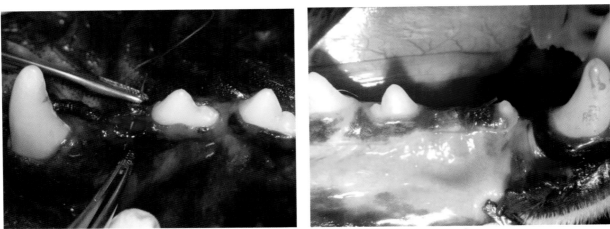

**Figure 19: Closure of the extraction site with simple interrupted suture.**

In regards to flap closure, there are several key points associated with successful healing.[2] The first and most important is there must be **no tension** on the incision line.[5,35,36] If there is any tension on the suture line, it will not heal. Tension can be removed by fenestrating the periosteum and/or extending the gingival incision along the arcade creating an envelope flap or by making vertical releasing incisions creating a full flap.[5,35-37] (see figure 20, 28, and 29 below)

16

The periosteum is a very thin fibrous tissue which attaches the buccal mucosa to the underlying bone.[40,41] Since it is fibrotic, it is inflexible and will interfere with the ability to close the defect without tension. The buccal mucosa is very flexible and therefore will stretch to cover large defects. If there is no tension, the flap should stay in position without sutures. Fenestration can be performed with a scalpel blade (a), however, LaGrange scissors offer more control (b). (Figure 20)

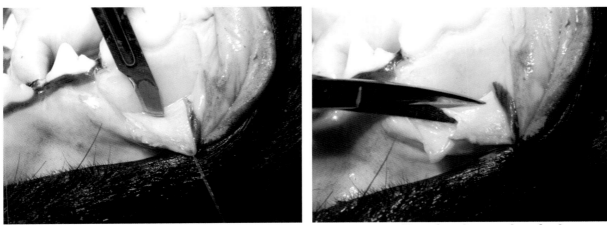

**Figure 20: Fenestration of the periosteum on a flap over the maxillary fourth premolar of a dog. This step can be performed with a scalpel (a) or scissors (b).**

If at all possible, the suture line should not be created over a void.[5,7] If sufficient tissue is present, consider removing some tissue on the attached side to make the suture line over bone.[35] Always suture from the unattached (flap side) to the attached tissue, in order to avoid tearing the flap as the needle dulls.[5] (Figure 21) Finally, ensure that all tissue edges have been thoroughly debrided, as intact epithelial tissues will not heal.[5] This is most important when closing an oronasal fistula.

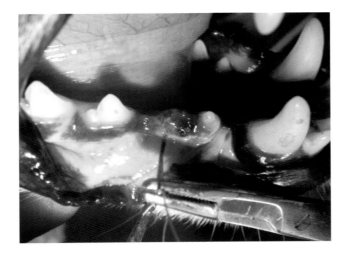

**Figure 21: Closing the defect from the buccal aspect first.**

## Step 10: <u>**EXPOSE A POST-OPERATIVE DENTAL RADIOGRAPH**</u>

Dental radiographs should be exposed post-extraction to document complete removal of the tooth.[1,10,42] (Figure 22) Retained roots are a very common complication associated with dental extractions. In fact, a recent study (accepted for publication in JAAHA) reported 92% of extracted carnassial teeth in dogs and cats have retained roots.

A retained root tip may become infected, or more commonly act as a foreign body creating significant inflammation.[2,43] There are rarely any clinical signs observed with this complication, but occasionally retained roots do create an abscess (and there have been some lawsuits levied over these cases).

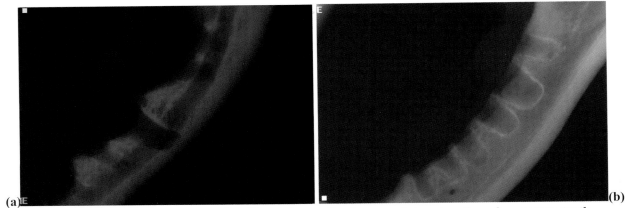

(a)                                                                                          (b)

**Figure 22 a: Post-operative dental radiographs confirming complete extraction of numerous teeth.**
**Mandibular premolars and molars in a dog (a) and cat (b).**

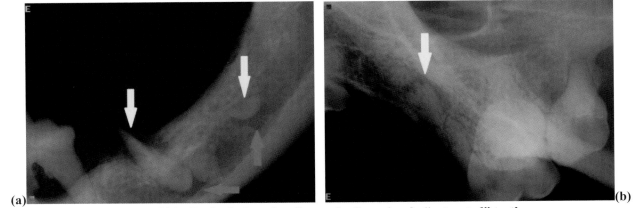

(a)                                                                                          (b)

**Figure 22 b: Recheck dental radiograph of previously "extracted" teeth.**
a) **Left mandibular first molar (309) of a dog with retained roots. (yellow arrows)**
**Note the jagged edge and alveolar bone loss on the mesial root.**
**Both root remnants have periapical rarefaction. (red arrows)**
**This tooth is infected despite the lack of clinical signs.**
b) **Left maxillary P4 (208) of a dog with a retained distal root. (yellow arrow)**
**This root also has associated rarefaction.**

## EXTRACTION OF MULTI-ROOTED TEETH

All multi-rooted teeth should be sectioned into single rooted pieces.[1,7,36] This is important because roots of most multi-rooted teeth are divergent (Figure 23), and thus the root tips will break if extractions are attempted in one piece.[2,9,37] Root fracture can occur even if a tooth is relatively mobile to start with. With mobile teeth, the sectioning step alone often allows for simple extraction.

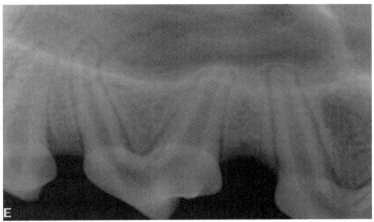

**Figure 23: Dental radiograph of the maxillary second premolar in a dog showing divergent roots.**

The best tool for sectioning teeth is a bur on a high-speed air driven hand piece.[1,5,36] In addition to being the most efficient tool, it also has air and water coolant to help avoid overheating the tooth and bone. Many different styles of burs are available. This author prefers a cross-cut taper fissure bur (699 for cats and small dogs, 701 for medium dogs, and 702 for large breeds).[2,3,5,7,9,36] When sectioning teeth, start at the furcation and work toward the crown.[2,5] (Figure 24) This method is used for two major reasons. First, it prevents the possibility of missing the furcation and cutting down into a root (which would weaken it and increase the risk of root fracture).[7] Second, this technique helps to avoid cutting through the tooth and inadvertently damaging the gingiva or alveolar bone.

If the furcation is not already exposed due to periodontal disease, a periosteal elevator should be used to carefully raise a small gingival flap to expose the furcation. Once the furcation is positively identified, sectioning can begin.

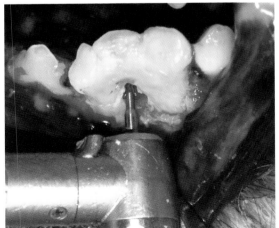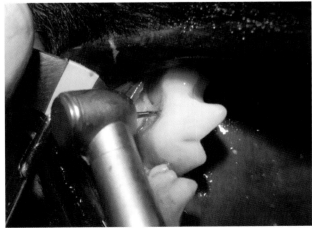

**Figure 24: Sectioning teeth with a 701 taper-fissure bur, starting at the furcation and advancing coronally.**

Two-rooted teeth are generally sectioned in the middle to separate the tooth into halves (Figure 25). The mandibular first molar in the cat is an exception, due to its disproportionate roots.

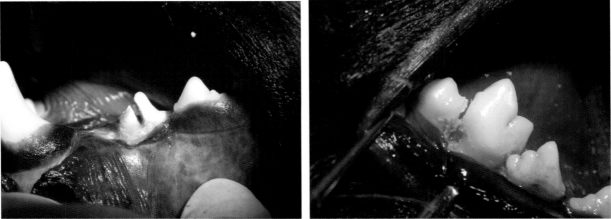

**Figure 25: A properly sectioned mandibular second premolar (left) and first molar (right) in a dog.**

Proper sectioning of a three-rooted molar tooth in a dog is performed by cutting between the buccal cusp tips and then just palatal to them. (Figure 26)

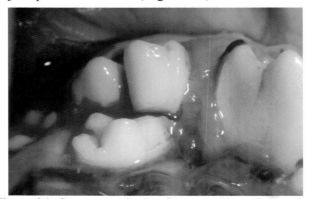

**Figure 26: Correct sectioning for a maxillary first molar.**

After the tooth has been properly sectioned, follow the previous outline of steps for each single rooted piece. In some cases, the individual tooth pieces can be carefully elevated against each other to gain purchase.[1 5 37] (Figure 27)

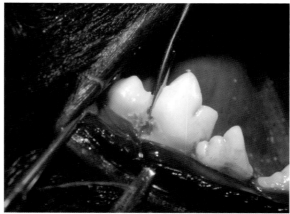

**Figure 27: Initial elevation between the two halves of a properly sectioned
two-rooted mandibular first molar.**

# SURGICAL EXTRACTIONS

Difficult extractions are best performed via a surgical approach.[9] This is typically utilized for the canine and carnassial (maxillary fourth premolar and mandibular first molar) teeth, but is also beneficial for teeth with root malformations or pathology and for retained roots.[1,5,6,7,35,37] With a surgical approach, buccal cortical bone can be removed promoting an easier extraction process. Surgical extractions are initiated by creating a gingival flap. Two options include a horizontal flap made with an incision along the arcade to create an **envelope flap** or alternatively making vertical releasing incisions to create a **full flap**.[1,5,35]

An envelope flap[44] is made by releasing the gingival attachment with a periosteal elevator along the arcade, including one to several teeth on either side of the tooth or teeth to be extracted.[9] (Figure 28) The flap is created by incising the gingiva in the interdental spaces along the arcade and then releasing the tissue to or below the level of the mucogingival junction (MGJ). Using this type of flap affords the advantage of not interrupting the blood supply and requiring less suturing for closure.

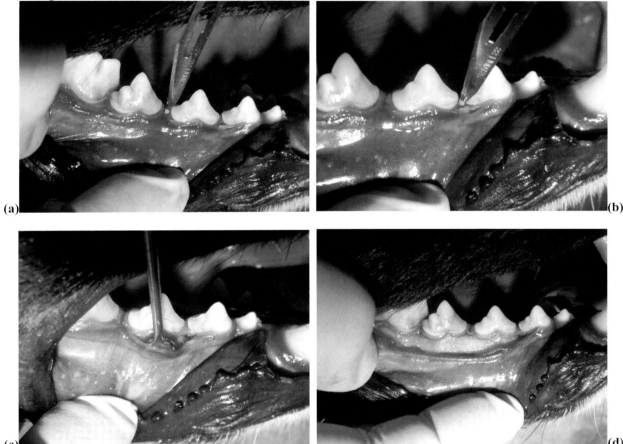

**Figure 28: Creation of an envelope flap.**
a & b)The interdental gingiva is incised between the teeth to be included in the flap.
Interdental incision made distal to the target tooth (a) and mesial to the target tooth (b).
The incision may extend to teeth which are not being extracted as long as the elevation is performed carefully.
c) The gingiva is carefully elevated with a periosteal elevator.
d) An envelope flap is created. Note, there is plenty of exposure for extraction and closure.

The more commonly used full flap includes one or two vertical releasing incisions.[1,3,37] (Figure 29) This method allows for a much larger flap to be created, which (if handled properly) means larger defects can be covered. Classically, the vertical incisions required to make this flap are made at the line angle of the target tooth, or one tooth mesial and distal to the target tooth.[7,36,45] Line angles are theoretic edges of teeth. However, if there is space between the teeth (either from a naturally occurring diastema or from previous extraction) the incision can be made in the space rather than extending to a healthy tooth. (Figure 30) (Small animal veterinary patients typically have natural space between their teeth, making these theoretic line angles more important in human dentistry.)

The vertical incisions for a full flap should be made slightly apically divergent, meaning wider at the base than at the gingival margin.[1,35-37] It is important to make full thickness incisions in one single motion (rather than performed with a slow and choppy motion). A full thickness incision is created by incising all the way to the bone, thus keeping the periosteum with the flap.[35-37] Once created, the entire flap is *gently* reflected with a periosteal elevator. Gentle handling is necessary to avoid tearing the flap, especially in cats or at the location of the mucogingival junction.

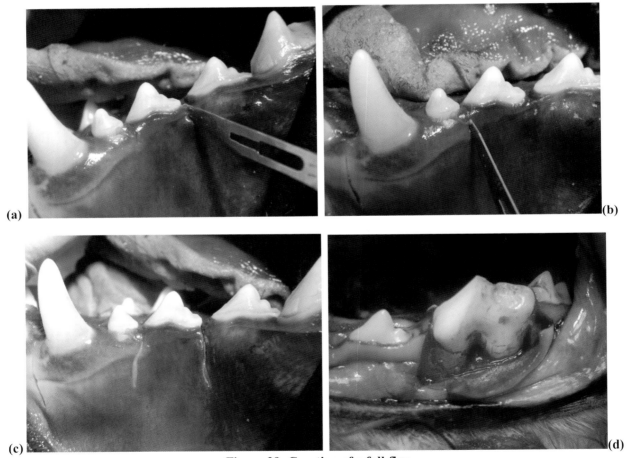

**Figure 29: Creation of a full flap.**
a) Making the distal releasing incision.
b) Creating the mesial releasing incision.
c) The slightly divergent releasing incisions.
d) Flap released over a maxillary fourth premolar on a clinical case.

22

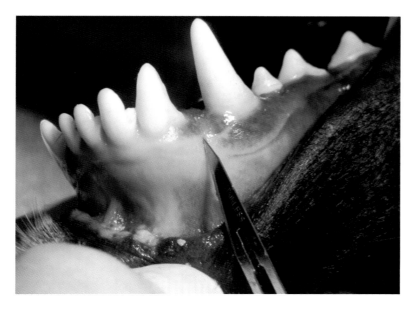

**Figure 30: Creating the mesial releasing incision for a maxillary canine extraction.**
**in the diastema between the canine and third incisor.**

Following flap elevation, buccal bone can be removed. (Figure 31) This author favors a cross cut taper fissure bur for this step. The preferred amount of buccal bone removal is controversial, with some dentists removing the entire buccal covering. This author prefers to maintain as much buccal bone as possible, starting with removal of an amount equal to 1/3 the root length of the subject tooth on the mandible or 1/2 the root length for maxillary teeth.[7,35] If this does not allow for extraction after an appropriate amount of time, more can be removed. If ankylosis is present, a significant amount of bone removal may be required. Bone removal should only be performed on the buccal side.

Following bone removal, multirooted teeth should be sectioned, and each piece removed as described in the steps previously outlined for single root extractions.[9] After the roots are removed and radiographic proof is obtained, the alveolar bone should be smoothed before closure (see alveoloplasty).

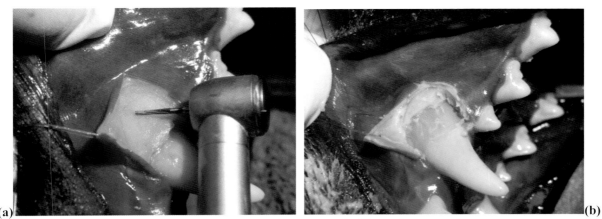

(a)                                                                                                          (b)

**Figure 31:  Removing buccal alveolar bone to facilitate the extraction process.**
**a) 701 crosscut taper fissure bur ready to remove bone from a maxillary canine.**
**b) Alveolar bone removed from the maxillary canine.**

Flap closure is initiated with an important step called "fenestrating the periosteum". The periosteum is a very thin fibrous tissue which attaches the buccal mucosa to the underlying bone.[41,44] Since the periosteum is fibrotic, it is inflexible and therefore interferes with the ability to close the defect *without* tension. The buccal mucosa however, is very flexible and will stretch to cover large defects. Consequently, incising the periosteum takes advantage of this attribute, making the flap more flexible. Fenestration should be performed at the base of the flap, and must be kept very shallow as the periosteum is very thin. This step requires careful attention in order to avoid cutting through or cutting off the entire flap. Fenestration can be performed with a scalpel blade, but a LaGrange scissors allows superior control.

After adequate fenestration, the mucogingival flap should stay in desired position without sutures. (Figure 32) If the flap does not remain in the desired position, tension is still present and further release is necessary prior to closure. Once adequate release is accomplished, the flap is sutured closed (as described above in the outlined closure step).

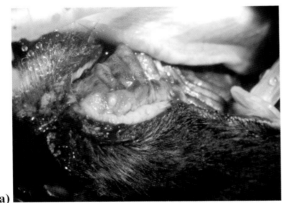 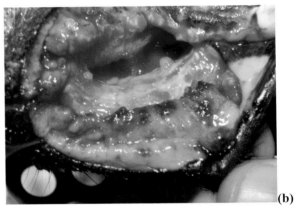

(a) (b)

**Figure 32: Pre-placement of the mucogingival flap to check for tension.**
a) **Flap stays in place without sutures.**
   **This is evidence that tension is released and healing should occur.**
b) **Flap pulls back.**
   **This shows that tension is present which means this flap would fail.**
   **Further tension release is required prior to closure.**

24

# MAXILLARY FOURTH PREMOLAR[36] (Figures 33 (dog) and 34 (cat))

Extraction of this tooth requires a gingival flap. Classically, this is a full flap with one or two vertical releasing incisons.[1,37] Full flaps provide good exposure and sufficient tissue for closure. However, this author finds envelope flaps sufficient for cats and small breed dogs.

**Full flaps** are created by making full thickness, slightly divergent incisions at the mesial and distal aspect of the tooth. (a)[7,36,37,45] Care should be taken to not damage the neighboring teeth. The flap incisions should be carried to a point just apical to the mucogingival junction. It is important to avoid cutting the infraorbital bundle as it exits the foramen above the third premolar. The flap is then gently elevated with a periosteal elevator.(b)

**Envelope flaps** are created by incising the interdental tissue between the tooth and the adjacent teeth.[9] The flap is then carefully elevated along the arcade, ensuring the gingiva over the teeth to be maintained is not damaged. (c)

Following flap creation (d), buccal bone is removed to a point approximately ½ the length of the root.(e) Next, the tooth is sectioned, separating mesial roots from the distal roots by starting at the furcation and cutting coronally. (f) The two mesial roots are then separated by sectioning in the depression between the palatal and buccal roots. (g) Another way to visualize this is to follow the ridge on the mesial aspect of the tooth. (h) A common mistake made during this step is not fully sectioning the tooth. The furcation is fairly deep, and must be fully sectioned in order to avoid root fracture. This can be confirmed by placing an elevator between the crown sections and twisting gently.(i) When fully sectioned, the pieces will move opposite each other easily. Following these steps, extraction proceeds as outlined above for single root pieces.

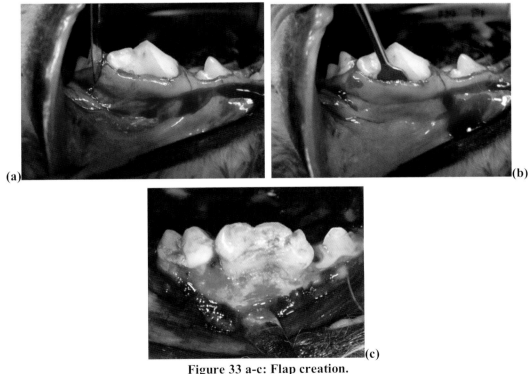

(a)

(b)

(c)

**Figure 33 a-c: Flap creation.**
**Images a & b: Full flap. Image c: envelope flap.**
**a) Distal vertical releasing incision (mesial incision already created).**
**b) Elevating the flap with a periosteal elevator.**
**c) Envelope flap created by incising gingiva from P3 to M1.**

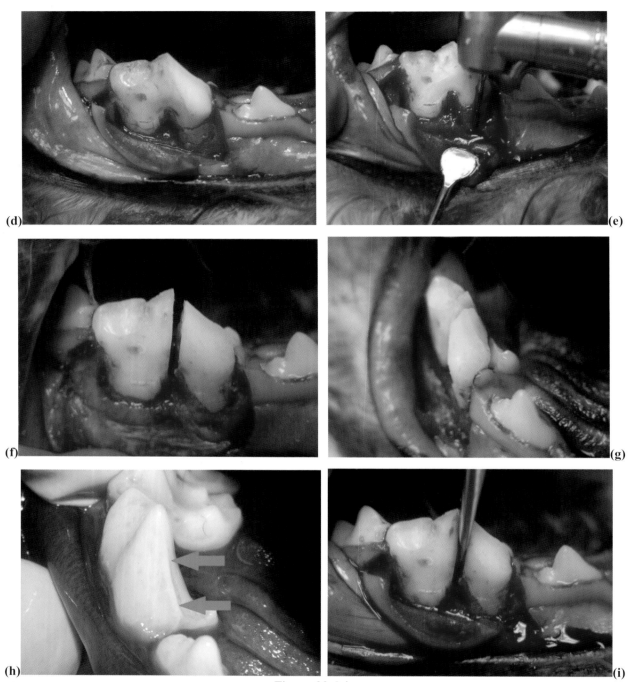

**Figure 33 d-i :**
d) "Full" flap elevated.
e) Removing buccal cortical bone with 701 bur.
f) Mesial roots sectioned from distal root.
g) Mesial roots sectioned.
h) Ridge on mesial aspect of this tooth leads to the furcation.
     Depicted with green arrows.
i) Using an elevator to ensure the tooth is fully sectioned.

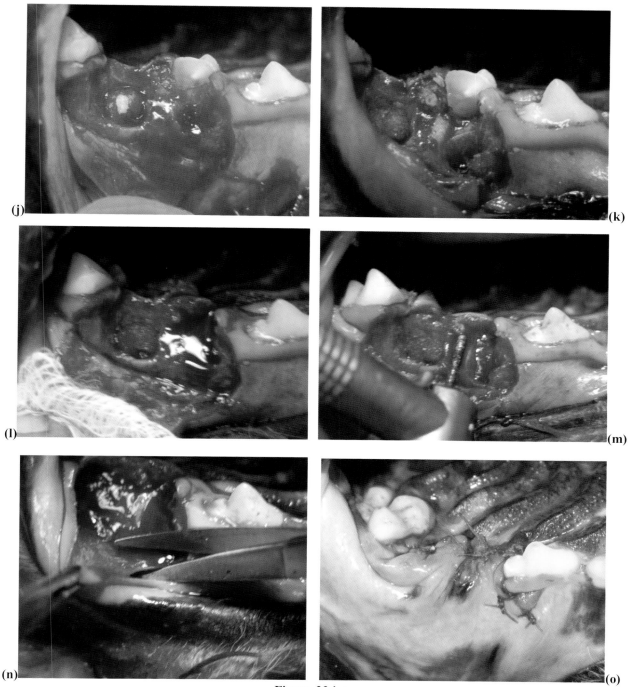

**Figure 33 j-o:**
j) Distal and mesio-buccal roots extracted.
k) Small amount of furcational bone removed over the palatine root to facilitate extraction.
l) The tooth is completely extracted.
m) Smoothing the alveolar bone and debriding the alveolus with a coarse diamond bur.
n) Fenestrating the periosteum with a LaGrange Scissors.
o) Closure with simple interrupted sutures.

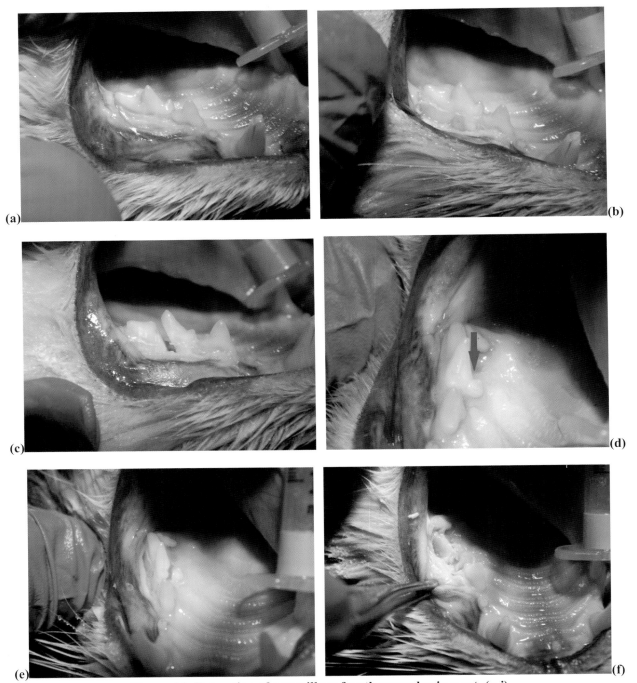

**Figure 34: Extraction of a maxillary fourth premolar in a cat. (a-i)**
a) Envelope flap created.
b) Buccal cortical bone removed.
c) Distal root sectioned from mesial roots.
d) "Trough" between mesial roots (blue arrow).
e) Mesial roots sectioned.
f) Tooth elevated and extracted.

28

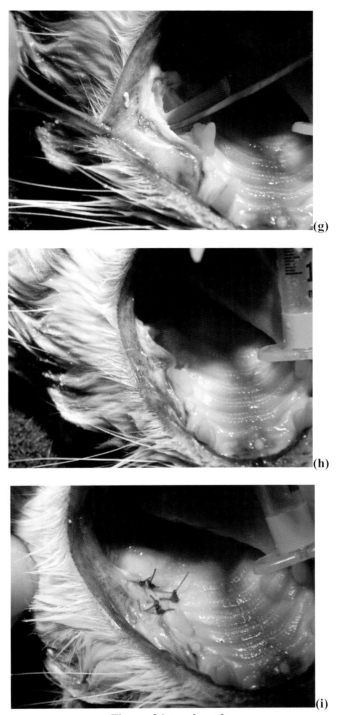

**Figure 34 continued:**
(g) Fenestrating the periosteum with a La Grange scissors.
(h) Ensuring there is no tension present before closure of flap.
(i) Closure is completed with just three sutures. (A major benefit of the envelope flap.)

# MANDIBULAR FIRST MOLAR[37] (Figure 35)

The mandibular first molar teeth are complicated extractions for many reasons. In dogs, the grooves on the furcational side of the roots of this tooth make elevation and root removal more difficult.[46] (a) In addition, the mesial root is often curved (b), and there may be a significant hook at the apex in small breed dogs.[9,10] (c) Furthermore, the roots of the mandibular first molar are much larger in proportion to the mandible in small and toy breeds as compared to larger breeds. Consequently, the roots reside within (and sometimes through) the mandibular canal (d), with minimal bone apical to the root,[10] which predisposes this area to pathologic mandibular fracture in small and toy breeds.[47] (e1 and e2) Periodontal disease and bony resorption can further weaken the bone and significantly add more risk of fracture in this area.[48] Finally, the mandibular nerve and vessels can be damaged during the extraction of the mandibular fist molar leading to significant hemorrhage.[13]

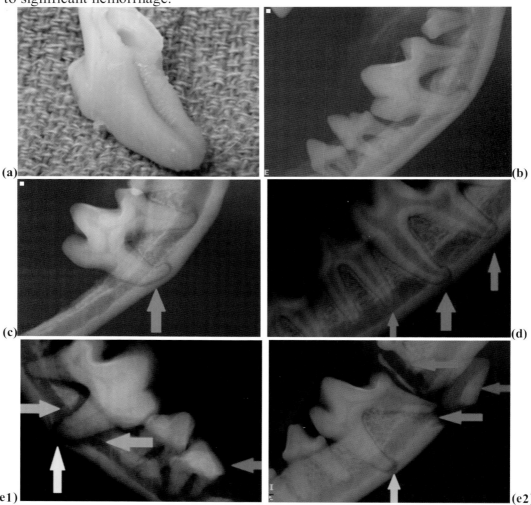

**Figure 35: Complications of mandibular first molar extractions.**
a) An extracted mesial root revealing the groove. b) Medium sized dog revealing a minor curve in the mesial root. c) Significant hook at the apex of the mesial root. (red arrow) d) Roots in and through the mandibular canal. e1) Severe vertical bone loss (blue arrows) and minimal (0.3 mm) ventral cortex (yellow arrows), predisposing to iatrogenic fracture. e2) Pathologic mandibular fracture at the distal root of the left mandibular first molar (309). (blue arrows). Also note the small area of periapical rarefaction on the mesial root (yellow arrow). Finally, there are free bone pieces (red arrow).

Pre-operative dental radiographs are required to demonstrate the level of remaining bone, in order to avoid iatrogenic damage. It is advised to warn clients of these potential complications with higher risk breeds. Referral to a dental specialist should be considered for these extractions, or for the option of root canal therapy.

The extraction procedure for the mandibular first molar generally requires a gingival flap. Classically, a full flap is utilized, with one or two vertical releasing incisions. However, this author finds that an envelope flap is sufficient in virtually all cases. (f)

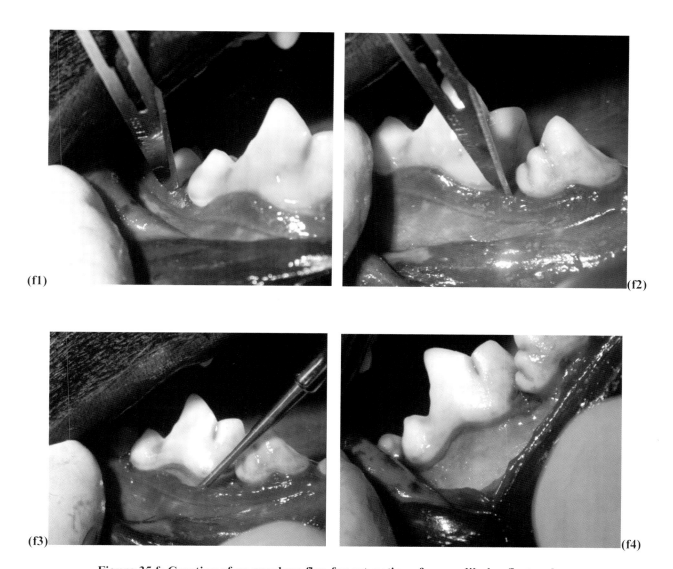

(f1)

(f2)

(f3)

(f4)

**Figure 35 f: Creation of an envelope flap for extraction of a mandibular first molar.**
1) Incising the interdental papilla between M1 and M2 (carried across M2).
2) Incising the interdental papilla between P4 and M1 (carried across P4).
3) Elevating the flap with a periosteal elevator.
4) Flap is created, and then held with a stay suture.

Following flap creation, buccal bone is removed to a point approximately 1/3 the length of the root. (g) More buccal bone can be taken if necessary. Next, the tooth is sectioned by starting at the furcation and cutting coronally. (h)

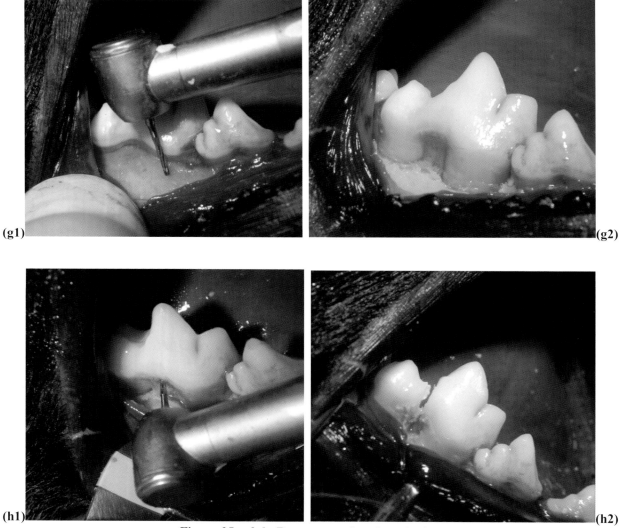

(g1)

(g2)

(h1)

(h2)

**Figure 35 g & h: Bone removal and sectioning.**

g1) **701 Surgical length bur poised to initiate bone removal.**
g2) **Buccal bone removed.**
h1) **Initiating sectioning at the furcation.**
h2) **Fully sectioned tooth, ready for elevation.**

Following these steps, extraction proceeds as outlined in the previous descriptions (i-l). The envelope flap should provide enough tissue for a tension free closure with minimal sutures.(m-n)

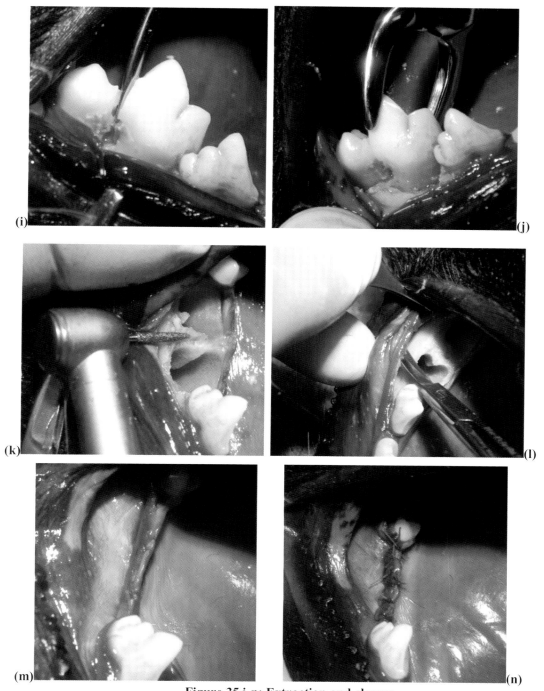

**Figure 35 i-n: Extraction and closure.**
i) Elevation.    j) Extraction.
k) Smoothing alveolar bone and debriding the alveolus with a coarse diamond bur.
l) Fenetrating the periosteum (blindly) with La Grange scissors.
m) Preplacing the flaps to ensure no tension is present.
n) Closure with 5 simple interrupted sutures.

The extraction of feline mandibular first molars is less complicated as the roots are much shorter. An important point for successful extraction of these teeth in cats is the discrepancy in root size. The distal root is very small, about 1/3 the size of the mesial root. (o) Therefore, the sectioning cut should be made about 2/3 of the way distally on the tooth. Creating a small gingival flap (p) in order to start the sectioning at the furcation ensures the position and angle of the cut will always be correct. (q) Furthermore, using small instruments in a very gentle manner will help to avoid fracturing this fragile root.

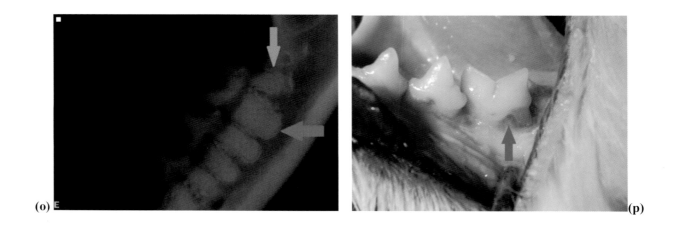

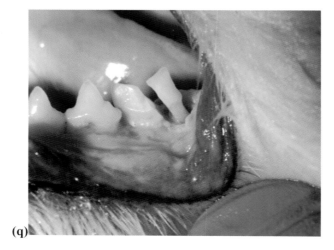

Figure 35 o-q: Anatomical variation of the feline M1.
o) Dental radiograph of the mandibular left of a cat. Note, the mesial root (red arrow) is significantly larger than the distal root (blue arrow).
p) Envelope flap created to expose the furcation. (blue arrow)
q) Properly sectioned mandibular first molar.

# MAXILLARY CANINE[35] (Figure 36)

Maxillary canines are very challenging extractions due to the significant length of the tooth root. (a) Furthermore, the plate of bone between the tooth root and the nasal cavity is very thin (less than 1-mm), creating a high risk of iatrogenic oronasal fistulas during extraction procedures.

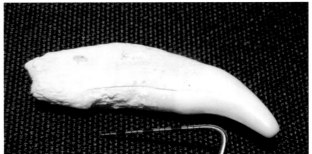

**Figure 36 a: Extracted canine tooth from a large breed dog.**
**The root is approximately 2.5 times longer than the crown.**
**The periodontal probe is provided for perspective.**

Mucogingival flaps made with vertical incisions are usually necessary for exposure as well as closure. At minimum, a distal incision should be performed, but adding a mesial incision creates more tissue available for closure.
The distal releasing incision is typically made at the mesial line angle of the first premolar.(b) An exception exists if the first premolar is very close to the canine. In this case, the mesial line angle of the second premolar is recommended. After the distal releasing incision is made, the interdental gingiva between the canine and first premolar is incised and the attached gingiva over the first premolar is carefully elevated. This should allow sufficient exposure for bone removal, as the root curves back over the second premolar.
Classically, the mesial incision was made at the mesial line angle of the canine tooth or distal line angle of the third incisor. However, in this author's opinion, the mesial line angle of the canine tooth does not allow sufficient exposure and there is no reason to risk damaging the third incisor and increasing surgical trauma. Therefore, if a mesial incision is performed, it should be made in the diastema between the canine and third incisor. (c)

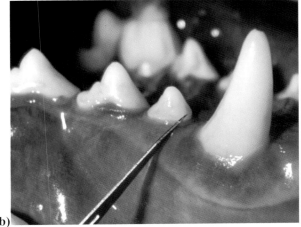
(b)
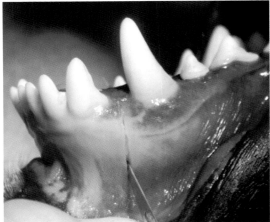
(c)

**Figure 36 b & c: Vertical releasing incisions for the maxillary canine.**
**b) Distal incision is initiated at the mesial line angle of the first premolar.**
**c) Mesial incision (optional) is created in the diastema between the canine and third incisor.**

It is critical to fully incise the interdental gingiva to avoid tearing the flap. (d) This is particularly challenging in the area mesial to the canine tooth. The incision must cut all the way to the bone.

After the vertical incisions are completed, the flap is carefully elevated. (e) If the flap cannot be elevated fairly easily, the interdental tissue is not fully incised, and this step should be repeated.

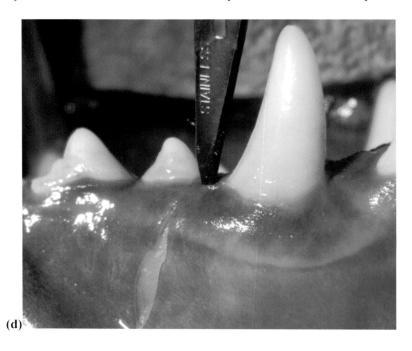

(d)

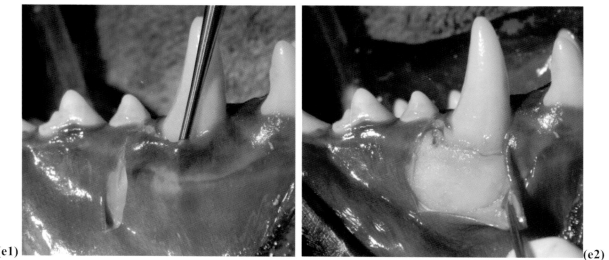

(e1)                                                                                             (e2)

**Figure 36 c & d: Flap creation (continued).**
**d) Incising the interdental gingiva to the level of the alveolar bone.**
**e1) Elevating the mucogingival flap with a periosteal elevator.**
**e2) Full thickness mucogingival flap created.**

Once the flap is raised, approximately ½ of the buccal bone should be removed. (f) It is important to remove some of the mesial and distal bone, as the tooth widens just under the alveolar margin.

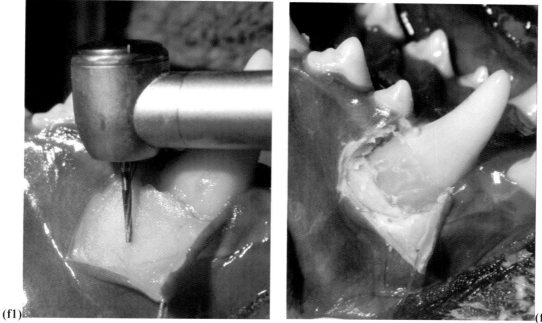

(f1)          (f2)

**Figure 36f: Buccal alveolar bone removal.**
**f1) Using a 701 surgical length bur to remove the buccal bone.**
**f2) Amount of bone removed equal to approximately ½ the root length.**
****Additional bone may be removed if necessary.**

After bone removal, the tooth is carefully elevated. (g) Caution must be used to avoid forcing the crown too much bucally, as this will lever the apex into the nasal cavity. Once the tooth is elevated to a point of very loose attachment, it can be carefully extracted with forceps. (h)

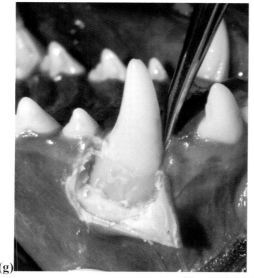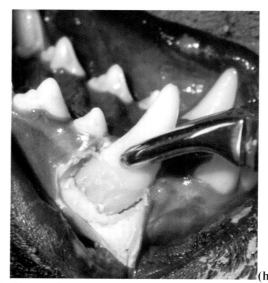

(g)          (h)

**Figure 36 g & h: Extraction**
**g) Careful elevation.**
**h) Extraction with forceps.**

Following extraction, the alveolus is debrided with a curette (i) and flushed. The alveolar bone is then smoothed with a coarse diamond bur. (j) Gingival closure is initiated with fenestration of the periosteum.[9] (k) After fenestration, the gingival tissue should stay in position over the defect. (l) If it does not, tension is present (and the flap will ultimately dehisce). It is critically important to relieve all tension if an oronasal fistula is present. Closure of the flap is done by placing the initial sutures at the corner(s) to ensure correct placement without tension. This step helps to avoid having to redo the entire closure if it does not place correctly to cover the defect after suturing most of it closed. After placing the corner sutures, the reminder of the incision is closed with simple interrupted sutures 2-3 mm apart. (m)

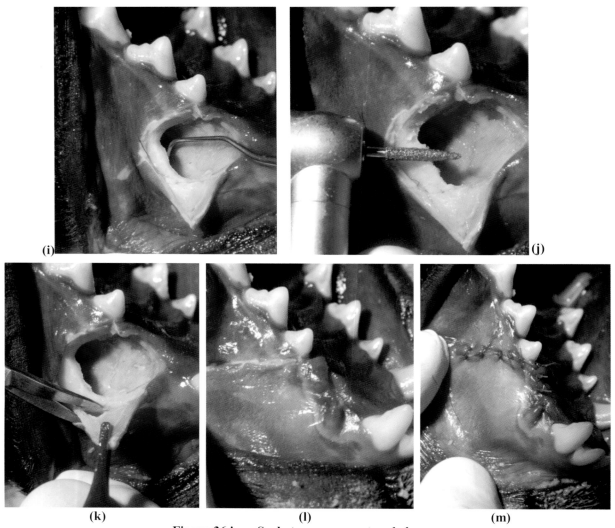

(i)　　(j)　　(k)　　(l)　　(m)

**Figure 36 i-m: Socket management and closure.**
i) Debriding the alveolus with a curette.
j) Smoothing the alveolar bone with a coarse diamond bur.
k) Fenestrating the periosteum with a La Grange scissors.
l) Placing the flap in position over the defect. If it stays in place, the tension is adequately released.
m) Closure is completed with simple interrupted sutures.

Regarding feline extractions, the only major difference is that the gingiva in cats is very thin and tightly attached to the bone. The horizontal incision is carried to the line angle of the second premolar (n1), and one distally divergent vertical incision is made to a point apical to the mucogingival junction.(n2) Following flap creation, the flap is *gently* elevated with a sharp periosteal elevator. (n3) Following extraction, the periosteum is *carefully* fenestrated at the base of the flap. (n4)

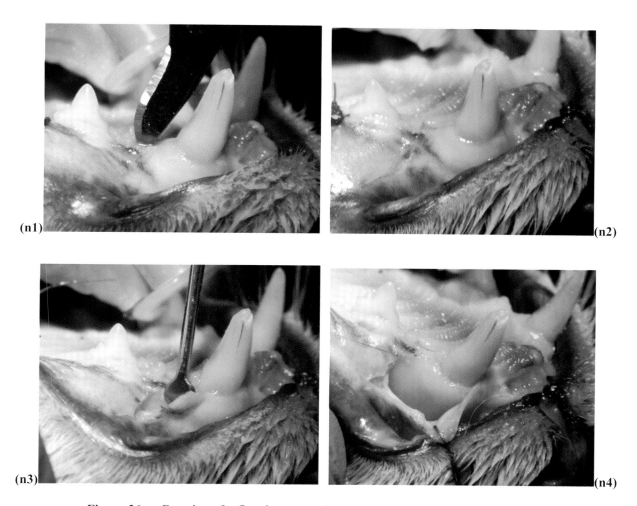

(n1)

(n2)

(n3)

(n4)

Figure 36 n: Creation of a flap for extraction of a maxillary canine tooth in a cat.
n1) Interdental incision between the canine and second premolar.
n2) Slightly divergent vertical incision starting at the mesial line angle of the second premolar.
n3) Careful elevation of the flap starting at the corner.
n4) Full thickness mucogingival flap created.

# MANDIBULAR CANINE (Figure 37)

These are quite simply the most difficult extraction in veterinary dentistry. There are several reasons for this, which include: the length and curve of the root (a), the hardness (i.e. less give) of the bone in the mandible, and the minimal amount of bone near the apex. (b) Furthermore, extraction of this tooth removes significant substance from the mandible leading to a weakened jaw which increases the risk of iatrogenic fracture either during or after surgery. It is important to note that the mandibular canine teeth hold the tongue in place within the mouth, and therefore it is not uncommon for the tongue to hang out following extraction of these teeth. Another disadvantage of this procedure is that the patient loses the function of this strategic tooth. For these numerous reasons, it is strongly recommended to avoid extraction of the mandibular canine teeth if possible, making referral for root canal therapy a much better option in many cases. Some authors recommend a lingual approach to this extraction since it requires less bone removal because the tooth root curves lingually as well as distally. However, this author prefers the standard buccal approach because superior exposure is afforded and the flexible buccal mucosa allows for an easier closure.

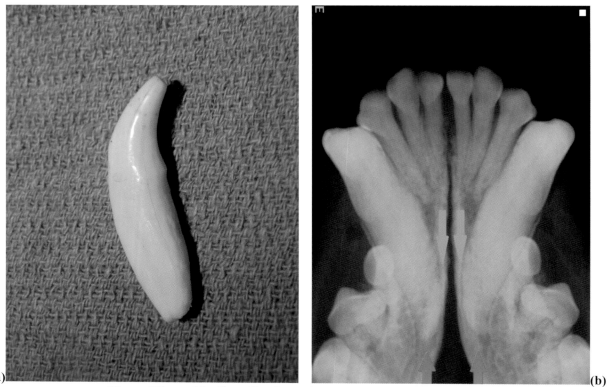

(a) (b)

**Figure 37 a and b: Complications of mandibular canine extraction.**
**a: Extracted mandibular canine tooth from a large breed dog showing the significant length of the root.**
**b: Dental radiograph of the mandibular canines in a dog. Note:**
- **The canines comprise the majority of the jaw structure in the area. (blue arrows)**
- **There is minimal bone apical to the canine teeth. (red arrows)**
- **The canine teeth are positioned more lingually nearer the apex.**

The best flap for mandibular canine tooth extraction is generally triangular with just one distal vertical incision. A horizontal incision is created along the arcade to the mesial line angle of the first premolar (c). Next, a distally divergent vertical incision is created. (d) The flap is then carefully elevated. (e)

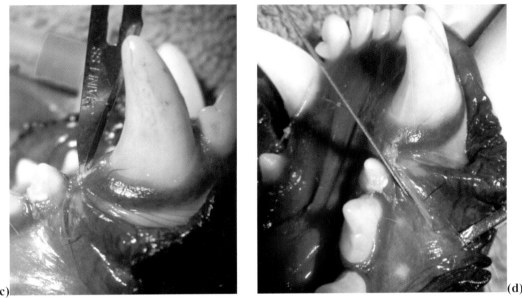

(c)                                                                                          (d)

**Figure 37 c & d: Flap incisions.**
**c) Horizontal incision between the canine and first premolar.**
**d) Slightly divergent vertical incision, started at line angle of the first premolar.**

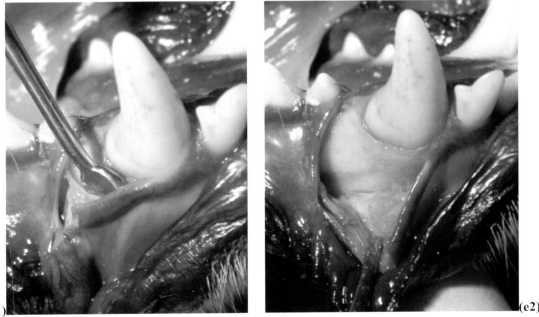

(e1)                                                                                        (e2)

**Figure 37 e 1 & 2: Elevating full thickness mucogingival flap.**
**e1) Careful elevation with a periosteal elevator.**
**e2) Flap created to expose buccal cortical bone.**

The buccal bone is then removed to a point approximately 1/3 of the way down the root. (f) More bone can be removed if necessary, but caution must be used when creating a larger flap or taking more bone, as the mental nerve and artery exit approximately 3/4 of the way down the root. Next, the tooth is carefully elevated and extracted. Care must be taken not to damage the third incisor or fracture the alveolar bone. It is helpful to use a small/sharp luxating elevator with gentle elevation.

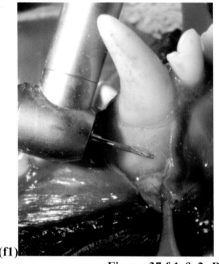 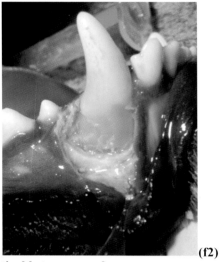

(f1)                                                   (f2)

**Figure 37 f 1 & 2: Buccal cortical bone removal.**
**f1) 701 taper fissure bur ready to remove bone.**
**f2) Enough bone is now removed to begin elevation.**

Gingival closure is initiated with fenestration of the periosteum.[9] (g,h) (See description above) After this is performed, the gingival tissue should stay in position over the defect. If it does not, tension is present and the flap will ultimately dehisce. The flap should be closed with the initial sutures placed at the corners to avoid having to redo the entire closure if it does not place correctly without tension.

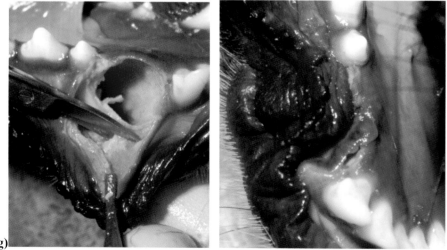

(g)                                                        (h)

**Figure 37 g: Careful fenestration of the periosteum with a La Grange scissors.**
**Figure 37 h: After fenestration, the flap stays in place, ensuring tension is released.**

Extraction of mandibular canine teeth in cats is very similar to that in dogs, except the gingiva is much more friable and the mandibular bone is thinner. In this case, the horizontal incision is carried to a point just mesial to the third premolar. (i) Following this, a slightly divergent vertical releasing incision is made at the line angle of the tooth. The flap is then gently elevated, taking the frenulum with it. (j) After flap creation, buccal bone is removed (k), and the tooth carefully elevated and extracted. The bone is smoothed and the periosteum fenestrated (as above). Preplace the flap to ensure that there is no tension present, (l) and close with simple interrupted sutures.

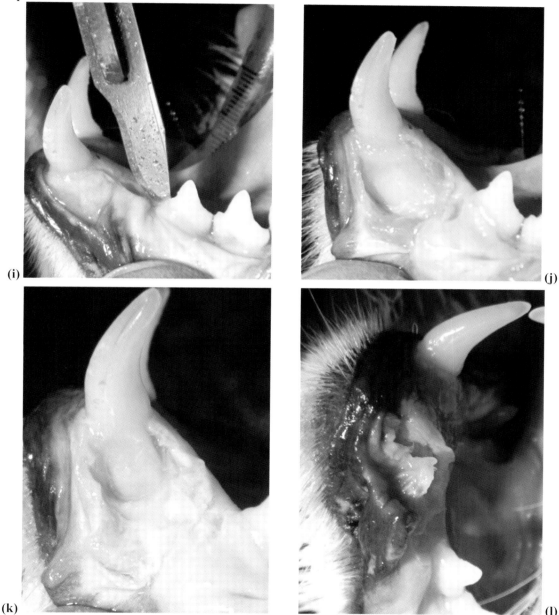

(i)

(j)

(k)

(l)

**Figure 37 i-l: Variation for extraction of a mandibular canine in a cat.**
**i) Creating horizontal incision between the canine and P3.**
**j) Gingival flap created and released.**
**k) Amount of buccal cortical bone removed is approximately 1/3 the root length.**
**l) Following fenestration, the flap should stay in position to confirm the lack of tension.**

# CROWN AMPUTATION[14,49]

The treatment of choice for teeth with tooth resorption (TRs) is extraction. However, crown amputation is an acceptable treatment option for advanced type 2 lesions. Crown amputation results in significantly less trauma to the patient and faster healing than complete extraction. This procedure, although widely accepted, is still controversial. Most veterinary dentists employ this technique, but opinions vary widely regarding the frequency of its use. Typically this treatment is chosen only when there is significant or complete root replacement by bone. Unfortunately however, the majority of general practitioners use this technique far too often.

Crown amputation can only be performed if certain criteria are met, which include: (Figure 38)

- Radiographically confirmed type 2 TRs
- No evidence of endodontic disease (periapical rarefaction)
- No evidence of periodontal bone loss
- No radiographically evident root canal
- No radiographic evidence of a periodontal ligament
- Caudal stomatitis is not present

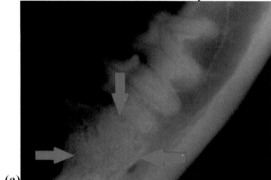
(a)
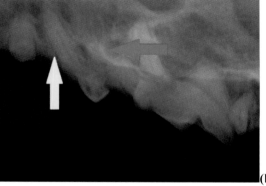
(b)

**Figure 38 a & b: Cases in which crown amputation would be appropriate.**
a) **Mandibular third premolar with complete bony replacement.**
**No periodontal ligament space or endodontic system is noted, and there is no evidence of bony lysis.**
b) **Maxillary third premolar with a mesial root which is normal and must be extracted (yellow arrow), but the distal root is resorbed and can be crown amputated (red arrow).**

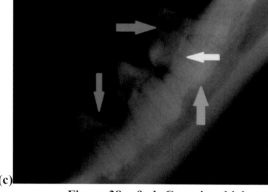
(c)
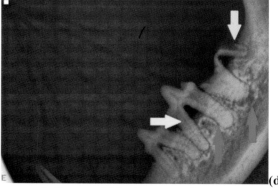
(d)

**Figure 38 c & d: Cases in which crown amputation would be inappropriate.**
c) **Advanced type 1 TRs (red arrows). There is significant tooth loss, but a normal appearing periodontal ligament space (blue arrow) and endodontic system (yellow arrow).**
d) **The fourth premolar has an early lesion, but a normal periodontal ligament space (purple arrow) and endodontic system (yellow arrow). The first molar has been incorrectly crown amputated and demonstrates periodontal bone loss (blue arrow) and periapical rarefaction (red arrow).**

44

This author tends to utilize this technique only for mandibular canines and third premolars. On occasion however, mandibular first molars (particularly the distal root) and maxillary canines may be treated in this manner. Other teeth can generally be extracted, regardless of radiographic findings.

Practitioners without dental radiology capability should NOT perform crown amputation. In these cases, the affected teeth should either be fully extracted or the patient referred to a facility with dental radiology.

**Crown Amputation Technique:** (Figure 39)
Once a suitable candidate has been found (a) and radiographically confirmed (see above), the procedure can begin. Crown amputation is initiated by creating a small gingival flap around the target tooth. (b-d) This is typically a conservative envelope flap.

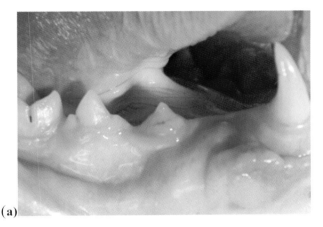
(a)

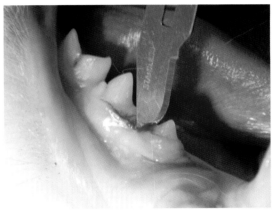
(b)

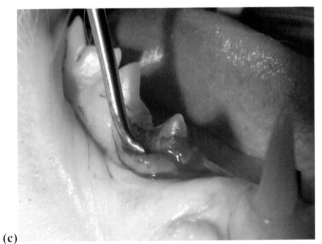
(c)

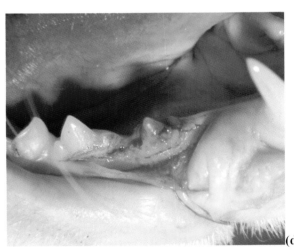
(d)

**Figure 39 a-d: Creation of the envelope flap.**
a)  A typical presentation of a tooth which is a candidate for crown amputation.
b)  Carefully incising the interdental gingiva between the P3 and P4.
    The incision is then carried along the tooth and approximately 5-mm mesial to the target tooth.
c)  Elevating the full thickness gingival flap with a periosteal elevator.
d)  Full thickness envelope flap created.

Next, a cross cut taper fissure bur on a high-speed handpiece is used to remove the entire crown to the level of the alveolar bone. (e) The bone and remaining tooth should be smoothed with a coarse diamond bur. (f)

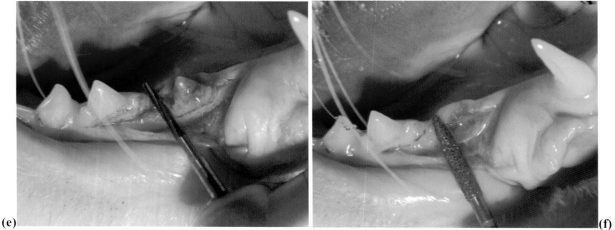

**Figure 39 e & f: Crown amputation.**
e) The crown is amputated with a # 701 crosscut taper fissure bur.
f) The bone is smoothed with a coarse diamond bur.

Following clinical (g) and radiographic confirmation that the tooth is removed to at least the level of the bone, the gingiva is sutured over the defect. (h) Closure may require a small amount of fenestration to relieve tension.

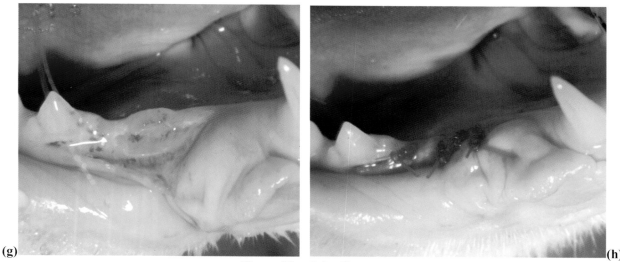

**Figure 39 g & h: Closure.**
g) Following crown amputation, the site is ready for closure.
h) Post-operative picture. Closure was achieved with only three sutures.

# EXTRACTION OF RETAINED ROOTS (Figure 40)

Root fracture is a very common problem in veterinary dentistry. The removal of retained root tips may seem to be a daunting task, but with proper technique and training, as well as the use of dental radiography, it can be fairly straightforward. The first step is to obtain radiographs to evaluate and visualize the retained roots. A gingival flap is necessary, and either an envelope flap (a) or a full flap (with one or two vertical releasing incisions) can be used depending on the anticipated amount of exposure required to retrieve the fragments. Following flap creation, buccal cortical bone is removed with a carbide bur to a point somewhat below the most coronal aspect of the remaining root. (b) If necessary, the bone can be removed 360 degrees around the tooth, but this author tries to avoid this aggressive approach. Once the root (s) can be visualized (c), careful elevation with small, sharp elevators is initiated. (d) Once the root is mobile, it can be extracted normally. After the root is extracted (e), the bone is smoothed and the defect closed.(f)

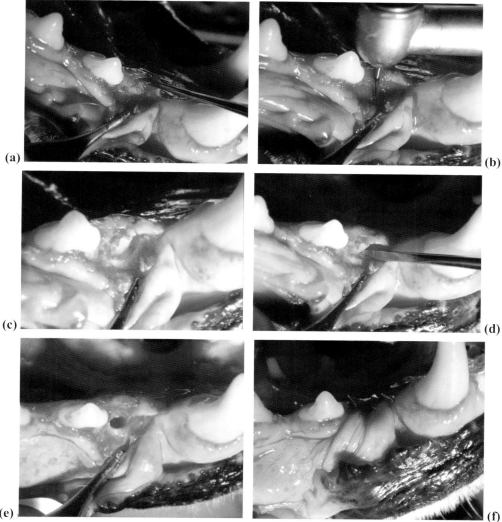

**Figure 40: Extraction of retained roots.**

| | |
|---|---|
| a) Creation of gingival flap (envelope). | b) Removal of buccal cortical bone. |
| c) Exposed root. | d) Elevation of exposed root. |
| e) Empty alveolus. | f) Closure of flap. |

# ORONASAL FISTULA REPAIR

## Robert B. Furman

An oronasal fistula (ONF) is defined as a communication between the oral and nasal cavities and occurs as a result of a defect in the gingival or palatal tissues and maxillary or incisive bone rostral to the third premolar.[2,50] Oroantral fistulas are defects distal to the third premolar.[50] Severe periodontal disease is the most common cause of acquired oronasal and oroantral fistulas in dogs.[50] Other causes of acquired fistulas include: trauma, neoplasia, iatrogenic associated with extractions (most commonly maxillary third incisors and canines), and burns from electrocution or caustic material.[51] The maxillary canine is the most common location of oronasal fistulas (Figure 41 a & b), but they can occur at any maxillary tooth.[2,50-54] (Figure 41 c & d) Several reparative techniques have been described, including: single layer flaps, double layer flaps, axial pattern flaps and autografts.[2,50-59]

In most cases, the single layer mucogingival flap technique is sufficient to repair ONFs, especially when done correctly the first time. This is the most common surgical treatment used to repair ONFs and therefore will be presented here.

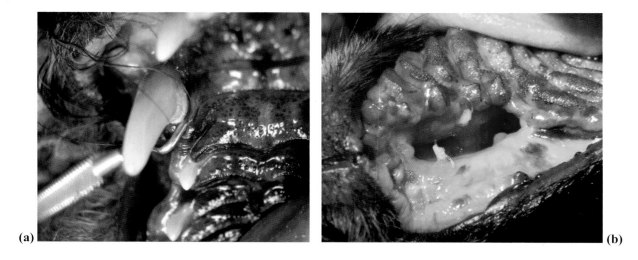

(a)  (b)

**Figure 41 a & b: Oronasal Fistulas at maxillary canine teeth:**
**(a) An oronasal fistula on the palatine surface of the right maxillary canine (104) of a dog.**
**Note, the tooth is present and there is minimal inflammation despite the severe disease to this tooth.**

**(b) Large oronasal fistula from the extraction site of the right maxillary canine (104) of a dog.**
**This patient had previous unsuccessful surgeries at a general practice.**
**(Note the remaining sutures from the prior repair attempts).**

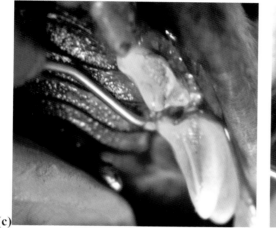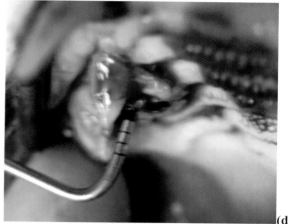

(c) (d)

**Figure 41 c & d: Oroantral fistulas at teeth other than canines.**
**c) Oroantral fistula on the palatal surface of the left maxillary fourth premolar (208) of a dog.**
**d) Oroantral fistula on the palatal surface of the right maxillary fourth premolar (108) of a cat.**

The single layer mucogingival flap is created with either one or two vertical incisions. Depending on the size and location of the fistula as well as presence of the offending tooth, a horizontal interdental incision may also be necessary for successful repair. Proper design of the mucogingival flap will allow maximum exposure of the area for extraction of the tooth (if necessary), debridement of the fistula, and a critically important tension-free closure.

Incisions are created with a number 15 or 11 scalpel blade. As described previously in the surgical extractions section, the vertical incision(s) are ideally started at the line angle of the teeth. A line angle is a theoretic corner of a tooth. When repairing an ONF associated with a maxillary canine tooth, the distal incision is made at the mesial line angle of the first premolar, and the mesial incision is started at the mesial line angle of the canine (if present). If the tooth is already absent, the incisions are made at the mesial and distal edges of the fistula.

The following images demonstrate repair techniques for an example case with the tooth still present, in comparison with an example case with the tooth already extracted. All images on the left (images marked **a**) depict repair of an ONF at the maxillary canine tooth of a cadaver. All images on the right (images marked **b**) depict a clinical case in which the tooth was already extracted. (Note, not all steps are imaged for the clinical case presentation.)

When making flap incisions, adequate pressure should be placed to ensure full thickness through the soft tissue which is incised down to the bone. The flap incisions should be created slightly divergent as they proceed apically, which allows for adequate blood supply to the newly created pedicle flap.[1,3,37] (Figure 42) It is important to choose the location of the incisions to ensure the sutured margins will have adequate bony support and will not lie over a defect. Alternatively, an incision can be made horizontally extending caudally one to two teeth, instead of a distal vertical incision. This results in a triangular shaped flap which decreases the risk of damaging blood supply (Figure 43).

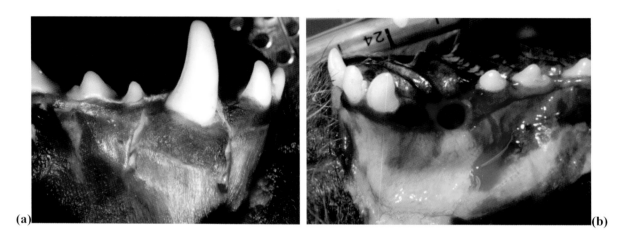

(a)                                                                                          (b)

**Figure 42 a & b: Mesial and distal vertical releasing incisions at the maxillary canine.**
**Note, the incisions are created slightly apically divergent.**

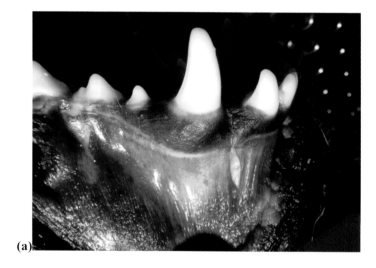

(a)

**Figure 43 a: Mesial vertical releasing incision to create a triangular flap.**
**This incision is slightly mesially divergent.**
**A horizontal incision has also been created back to the level of the second premolar.**

The mucogingival flap is gently elevated off the bone using a periosteal elevator (Figure 44). (If the tooth is present, it is extracted as described in previous sections).

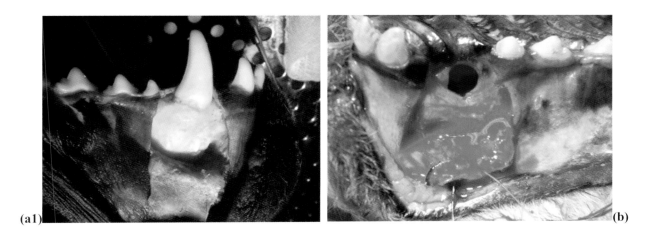

(a1)                                                                                          (b)

**Figure 44 a1 & b: Both cases demonstrate full flaps with 2 vertical releasing incisions.**

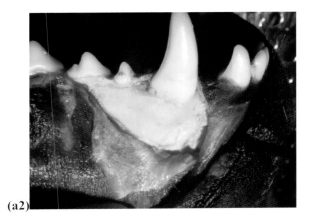

(a2)

**Figure 44 a2: This image demonstrates a single (mesial) releasing incision for a triangular flap.**

Approximately 2-3mm of palatal mucosa is also gently elevated/lifted off the palatal bone in order to create fresh epithelial edges. Any margins of the flap which are associated with the oronasal fistula should be debrided using a LaGrange scissors or coarse diamond bur, removing 1-2mm of tissue, and therefore leaving fresh epithelial edges.

A coarse diamond bur on a high-speed handpiece is used to smooth the edges of the remaining maxillary bone (if necessary) and to remove any epithelial remnants between the fistula and the nasal cavity. (Figure 45)

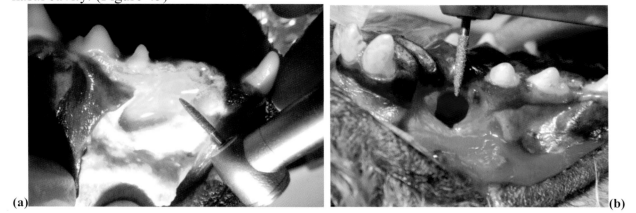

(a)                                                                                                      (b)

**Figure 45 a & b: Smoothing alveolar bone and debriding necrotic tissue.**
**a) Smoothing the bony edges with a coarse diamond bur on a high-speed hand-piece.**
**b) Debriding the epithelium with a coarse diamond bur on a high-speed hand-piece.**

As with any closure in the oral cavity, the key to success is to ensure there is no tension on the incision line. Fenestration of the inelastic periosteum (see previous section on surgical extractions) is performed to increase the mobility of the flap and allow for a tension free closure. This is accomplished by a combination of sharp and blunt dissection with a LaGrange scissors while ensuring the overlying mucosa is not damaged. (Figure 46)

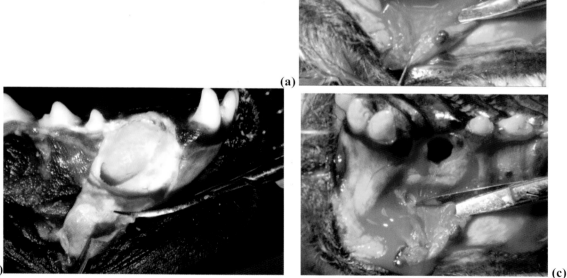

(a)

(b)                                                                                                      (c)

**Figure 46 a-c: Careful fenestration of the periosteum with LaGrange scissors.**
**a: Careful undermining of the periosteum to release from the buccal mucosa.**
**b & c: Cutting the elevated periosteum.**

52

The gingival flap is then placed over the defect so that it remains in position without being held. Once this is accomplished (i.e. no tension is present), the flap is ready to be sutured into place. (Figure 47) If the flap pulls back at all, tension is present and must be released prior to closure.

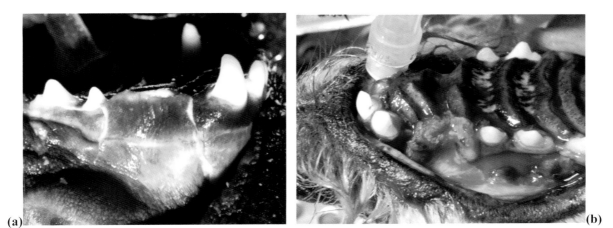

(a)                                                                                                    (b)

**Figure 47 a & b: The flap is placed in the desired position and released.
Note, the flap stays in position, which indicates that tension is released and closure can begin.**

Placing a second (buried) layer can improve the chances of healing. A few buried horizontal mattress sutures will help maintain the flap as well as smooth out the incision line. (Figure 48) Furthermore, this layer cannot be easily removed by the patient.

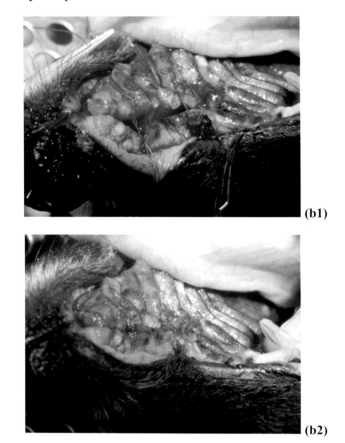

**(b1)**

**(b2)**

**Figure 48 b 1 & 2:  Two-layer closure.**
**b1) Preplaced horizontal mattress sutures which will be "buried" when tied.**
**b2) After placement of the horizontal mattress sutures, the flap is already held well in position.**

Closure is performed as described in previous sections. The initial sutures are placed at the corners of the flap to avoid having to resuture the flap if it does not align correctly. (Figure 49a) This is not necessary if a subcuticular layer has been placed.

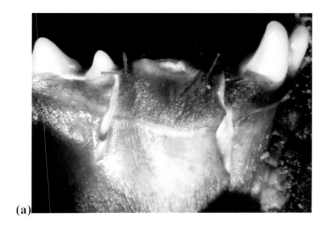
(a)

**Figure 49 a: Corners have been sutured in place, in order to determine the flap is well sized and positioned.**

Once it has been determined that the flap properly fits the defect, the remaining edges are sutured closed. This is done in a simple interrupted pattern, placing sutures 2-3 mm apart. (Figure 50) Suture lines should always be placed over bone, avoiding placement over empty space which was created by tooth/bone removal.

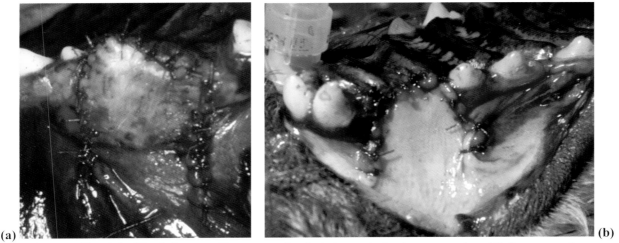
(a)                                                                (b)

**Figure 50 a & b: Final closure. Numerous simple interrupted sutures are placed 2-3 mm apart.**

# DECIDUOUS TOOTH EXTRACTION

Deciduous tooth extraction is very similar to the process used for permanent dentition with a few notable exceptions. The steps are essentially performed as outlined for simple extractions above. Much of the current literature recommends closed extractions in cases with significant root resorption and a surgical approach when the tooth appears intact.[32,43] However, many veterinary dentists (including this author) prefer the simple or closed technique for the majority of deciduous extractions due to decreased surgical time and trauma.[3,60] Surgical extractions of deciduous canines are accomplished by performing gingival flaps and buccal bone removal as shown in figures 36 and 37.

There are several subtle differences between deciduous and permanent dentition which can make deciduous extractions challenging. First, deciduous roots are proportionally much longer than the corresponding permanent dentition.[3,61] (Figure 51) Furthermore, deciduous teeth have very thin walls making them more susceptible to fracture.[60] Natural root resorption of deciduous teeth, which occurs as a result of pressure from the erupting permanent tooth as well as normal aging, can complicate extractions. Finally, deciduous extractions must be done with caution to avoid damaging the developing permanent tooth.[32,43,60]

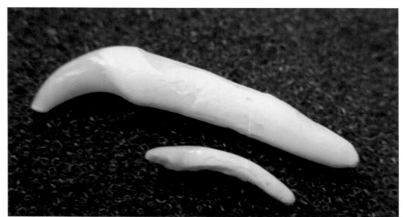

**Figure 51: Extracted deciduous canine and incisor from a dog.**
**The roots of these teeth are approximately 5 times the length of the crown.**

Dental radiographs are critical to document the presence (or absence) of the permanent dentition, and to reveal the location and integrity of the permanent teeth.[10,60,61] Radiographs will also reveal the root structure of the deciduous teeth, which is important for procedure planning. It is important to know if the root resorption is partial or complete (Figure 52), in order to avoid unnecessary exploration for a previously resorbed root or leaving a retained root in place. Furthermore, while complete root resorption may simplify the extraction procedure, partial root resorption tends to make it more difficult due to the weakened area creating a higher risk for root fracture.

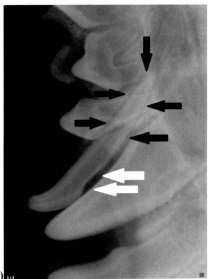 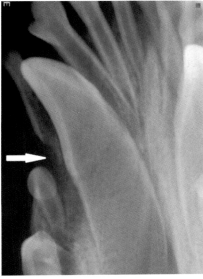

(a)                                                                              (b)

**Figure 52: The importance of pre-operative dental radiographs for deciduous extractions.**
**a) The erupting permanent maxillary canine created an area of resorption on the neck of the persistent deciduous (white arrows). This will greatly increase the likelihood of fracture, if care is not taken in the extraction attempt. However, the apical area of the root is normal (black arrows) and requires complete extraction. A surgical approach is advised in this case.**
**b) This persistent mandibular canine root is completely resorbed and held in place by the attached gingiva. Simple extraction of the crown is all that is required.**

Deciduous tooth extraction must be performed carefully, gently, and patiently. Only very small (1-2 mm) luxating elevators should be used for deciduous tooth extractions. The instrument is inserted into the periodontal ligament space and gentle pressure used for elevation. Extra caution is required when performing elevation if the permanent tooth has not yet erupted. Finally, it is important to avoid deep elevation on the aspect where the permanent tooth will erupt (i.e. distal aspect of the deciduous maxillary canine and lingual aspect of the mandibular canine).
Root fractures are common complications of deciduous extraction attempts. If this occurs, every effort should be made to remove the retained piece(s).[2,32,60] A retained root tip may become infected, or more likely act as a foreign body, creating significant inflammation.[2, 43,60] Unfortunately for animal patients, clinical signs are rarely seen, but retained roots **are** painful and/or infected. Complete root tip removal is even more critical when performed for certain interceptive orthodontic purposes (especially linguoclused mandibular canines), because the tip alone is sufficient to deflect the permanent tooth from its normal eruptive path.[2,60] Retained roots are best extracted utilizing a surgical approach.[3,32,60]
Post-operative dental radiographs are strongly recommended following extraction, in order to prove complete removal of the deciduous tooth as well as the presence and proper condition of the unerupted permanent teeth.

# CONCLUSION

Extractions are a very common procedure in veterinary medicine, but at times can be complicated and therefore very frustrating for the practitioner. If extractions are performed correctly, this treatment is an excellent means to alleviate oral pain and infection. However, if extraction procedures are not planned or performed appropriately, they can and will result in problems such as fractured root tips and/or more serious iatrogenic complications. Appropriate planning includes scheduling adequate time for dental procedures as for an any other surgical procedure. It also includes obtaining sufficient knowledge and training for these specific skills and procedures. Furthermore, the performance of extractions requires utilization of proper equipment which is also appropriately maintained. Additionally, it is critical to remember that PATIENCE is of utmost importance in successful dental extractions. Once these essentials are in place, practitioners can use the guidelines and outlined steps provided here to facilitate extractions and improve outcome and overall sucess.

This is a win-win situation for the practitioner and the patient.

# KEY POINTS

- Hands-on laboratories are a valuable learning tool and will greatly benefit practitioners and their patients.
  - www.dogbeachvet.com
- Extractions are surgical procedures and must be treated with the same level of respect as any other surgery in order to avoid complications.
- All extractions can be made into simple, single root extractions via sectioning and buccal cortical bone removal. Therefore, any extraction can be performed once the basic skills are mastered.
- Extractions are painful procedures which require appropriate pain management, including regional anesthesia (nerve blocks).
- Crown amputation is an accepted method of therapy specifically for advanced **type 2** lesions in cats and only if certain criteria (clinical and radiographic) are met.
- Never extract a tooth without client consent.

# REFERENCES

[1] Holmstrom SE, Frost P, Eisner ER: Exodontics, in Veterinary Dental Techniques (2 ed). Philadelphia, PA, Saunders, pp. 238-42, 1998.

[2] Wiggs RB, Lobprise HB: Oral Surgery, in Veterinary Dentistry, Principals and Practice. Philadelphia, PA Lippincott – Raven, pp. 312-77, 1997.

[3] Harvey CE, Emily PP: Oral Surgery. In Small Animal Dentistry. Mosby, St. Louis, pp. 213-65, 1993.

[4] Taylor TN, Smith MM, Snyder L: Nasal displacement of a tooth root in a dog. J Vet Dent. 21(4):222-5, 2004.

[5] Blazejewski S, Lewis JR, Reiter AM: Mucoperiosteal flap for extraction of multiple teeth in the maxillary quadrant of the cat. J Vet Dent. 23(3): 200-5, 2006.

[6] Woodward TM: Extraction of fractured tooth roots. J Vet Dent. 23(2): 126-9, 2006.

[7] Smith MM: Exodontics. In: Vet Clin N Am Sm Anim Pract. 28(5): 1297-1319, 1998.

[8] Shipp AD, Fahrenkrug P: Exodontics, In Practitioner's Guide to Veterinary Dentistry. Dr. Shipp's Laboratories, Beverly Hills, pp. 60-65, 1992.

[9] Niemiec BA: Extraction Techniques. Top Companion Anim Med. 23(2):97-105, 2008.

[10] Niemiec BA: Case Based Dental Radiology. Top Companion Anim Med. 24(1):4-19, 2009.

[11] Verstraete FJ, Terpak CH: Anatomical Variation in the Dentition of the Domestic Cat. J Vet Dent.14 (4): 137-40, 1997.

[12] Mulligan T, Aller S, and Williams, C: Atlas of Canine and Feline Dental Radiography. Trenton, New Jersey, Veterinary Learning Systems, pp. 176-83, 1998.

[13] Gioso MA, Shofer F, Barros PS, Harvey CE: Mandible and mandibular first molar tooth measurements in dogs: relationship of radiographic height to body weight. J Vet Dent. 18(2): 65-8, 2001.

[14] DuPont G: Crown amputation with intentional root retention for advanced feline resorptive lesions: a clinical study. J Vet Dent. 12(1):9–13, 1995.

[15] Kelly DJ, Ahmad M, Brull SJ: Preemptive analgesia I: physiological pathways and pharmacological modalities. 48(10):1000-10, 2001.

[16] Kelly DJ, Ahmad M, Brull SJ: Preemptive analgesia II: recent advances and current trends. Can J Anesth. 48(11):1091-101, 2001.

[17] Lanz GC: Regional Anesthesia for Dentistry and Oral Surgery. J Vet Dent. 20(3): 181-6, 2003.

[18] Woodward TM: Pain Management and Regional Anesthesia for the Dental Patient. Top Companion Anim Med. 23(2):106-14, 2008.

[19] Sawyer DC, Rech RH, Durham RA, Adams T, Richeter MA, Striler EL: Dose response to butorphenol administered subcutaneously to increase visceral nociceptive threshold in dogs. Am J Vet Res. 52(11):1826-30, 1991.

[20] Holmstrom SE, Frost P, Eisner ER: Anesthesia and Pain Management in Dental and Oral Procedures. In: Veterinary Dental Techniques (Ed 2). Philadelphia, PA, Saunders. pp. 481-96, 1998.

[21] Mama KR: Local Anesthetics. In: Handbook of Veterinary Pain Management (Ed 2). (Gaynor JS, Muir WW eds). St. Louis: Mosby, pp. 231-48, 2008.

[22] Gross R, McCartney M, Reader A, Beck M: A prospective, randomized, double-blind comparison of bupivacaine and lidocaine for maxillary infiltrations. J Endod. 33(9):1021-4, 2007.

[23] Lai F, Sutton B, Nicholson G: Comparison of L-bupivacaine 0.75% and lidocaine 2% with bupivacaine 0.75% and lidocaine 2% for peribulbar anesthesia. Br J Anaesth. 90(4):512-4, 2003.

[24] Valvano M, Leffler S: Comparison of Bupivacaine and Lidocaine/Bupivacaine for Local Anesthesia/Digital Nerve Block Ann Emerg Med. 27(4): 490-2, 1996.

[25] Lee-Elliott CE, Dundas D, Patel U: Randomized trial of lidocaine vs. lidocaine/bupivacaine periprostatic injection on longitudinal pain scores after prostate biopsy. J Urol. 171(1):247-50, 2004.

[26] Kaukinen S, Kaukinen L, Eerola R: Epidural anesthesia with mixtures of bupivacaine-lidocaine and etidocaine-lidocaine. Ann Chir Gynaeco. l69(6):281-6, 1980.

[27] Shama T, Gopal L, Shanmugam MP, et al: Comparison of pH-adjusted bupivacaine with a mixture of non-pH-adjusted bupivacaine and lignocaine in primary vitreoretinal surgery. Retina. 22(2): 202-7, 2002.

[28] Mama K: Local anesthetics. In: Handbook of Veterinary Pain Management (Gaynor JS, Muir WW eds). St. Louis, Mosby, pp. 221-39, 2002.

[29] Bazin JE, Massoni C, Bruelle P, Fenies V, Groslier D, Schoeffler P: The addition of opioids to local anesthetics in brachial plexus block: the comparative effects of morphine, buprenorphine and sufentanil. Anesthesia. 52(9):858-62, 1997.

[30] Beckman, BW: Pathophysiology and management of surgical and chronic oral pain in dogs and cats. J Vet Dent. 23(1):50-60, 2006.

[31] Evans HE, Christensen GC: Miller's Anatomy of the Dog, 2nd Ed, Saunders, Philadelphia. pp. 914-20, 1997.

[32] Hobson P: Extraction of retained primary teeth in the dog. J Vet Dent 22(2): 132-7, 2005.

[33] Smith MM, Smith EM, La Croix N, Mould J: Orbital penetration associated with tooth extraction. J Vet Dent. 20(1): 8-17, 2003.

[34] Proffit WR, Fields HW: Contemporary Orthodontics (Ed 3). St. Louis, Mo, Mosby. pp. 297-306, 2000.

[35] Frost Fitch P: Surgical extraction of the maxillary canine tooth. J Vet Dent. 20(1): 55-8, 2003.

[36] Carmichael DT: Surgical extraction of the maxillary fourth premolar tooth in the dog. J Vet Dent. 19(4): 231-3, 2002.

[37] Manfra Marretta S: Surgical extraction of the mandibular first molar tooth in the dog. J Vet Dent. 19(1):46-50, 2002.

[38] Taney KG, Smith MM: Surgical extraction of impacted teeth in a dog. J Vet Dent. 23(3): 168-77, 2006.

[39] Wilson J, Clark AE, Hall M, Hench LL: Tissue response to Bioglass endosseous ridge maintenance implants. J Oral Implantol, 19(4):295-302, 1993.

[40] Evans HE: The skeleton, in Miller's anatomy of the dog (3rd Ed) Philadelphia, PA, W.B. Saunders. pp. 122-218, 1993.

[41] Grant DA, Stern IB, Listgarten MA: Alveolar Process. In, Periodontics. St. Louis, MO, C.V. Mosby. pp. 94-118, 1988.

[42] Holmstrom SE, Bellows J, Colmrey B, Conway ML, Knutson K, Vitoux J: AAHA dental care guidelines for dogs and cats. J Am Anim Hosp Assoc 41, 2005.

[43] Ulbricht RD, Marretta SM, Klippert LS: Surgical Extraction of a Fractured, Nonvital Deciduous Tooth in a Tiger. J Vet Dent. 20(4): 209–12, 2003.

[44] Grant DA, Stern IB, Listgarten MA: Periodontal flap. In, Periodontics. St. Louis, MO, C.V. Mosby. pp. 786-822, 1988.

[45] Smith MM: Line angle incisions. J Vet Dent. 20(4): 241-44, 2003.

[46] Woodward TM: Interpretation of dental radiographs. Top Companion Anim Med. 24(1):37-43, 2009.

[47] Niemiec BA: Periodontal disease. Top Companion Anim Med. 23(2):72-80, 2008.

[48] Mulligan T, Aller, S, Williams C: Atlas of Canine and Feline Dental Radiography. Trenton, New Jersey, Veterinary Learning Systems. pp. 176-83, 1998.

[49] Bellows J: Treatment of Tooth Resorption. In: Feline Dentistry: Oral Assessment, Treatment, and Preventative Care. Wiley Blackwell, Ames Iowa, pp. 222-41, 2010.

[50] Niemiec BA: Problems with the oral mucosa. In: Small Animal Dental Oral & Maxillofacial Disease (Niemiec BA (Ed)). Manson Publishing, London, pp. 183-98, 2010.

[51] Smith MM: Oronasal fistula repair. In, Clin Techniques, Sm Anim Pract. 15(4):243-50, 2000.

[52] Fossum TW, Hedlund CS, Johnson AL, et al: Small Animal Surgery. Mosby Elsevier, St. Louis. pp. 356-61, 2007.

[53] Bellows J: Small Animal Dental Equipment, Materials and Techniques. Blackwell Publishing, Ames, Iowa, pp. 157-158, 2004.

[54] Holmstrom SE: Oronasal-Oroantral Fistulas. In: Vet Clin N Am Sm Anim Pract. 28(5): 1289

[55] Soukup JW, Snyder CJ, Gengler WR: Free Auricular Autograft for Repair of an Oronasal Fistula in a Dog. J Vet Dent. 26(2):86-95, 2009.

[56] Manfra Marreta SM, Smith MM: Single Mucoperiosteal Flap for Oronasal Fistula Repair. J Vet Dent 22(3):200-5, 2005.

[57] Woodward TM: Greater Palatine Island Axial Pattern Flap for Repair of Oronasal Fistula Related to Eosinophilic Granuloma. J Vet Dent. 23(3):161-6, 2006.

[58] Wetering A, Caldwell L, Loman S, Reid T: Repair of Palatal Oronasal Fistulae Using Auricular Cartilage Graft. J Vet Dent. 27(2):128-31, 2012.

[59] Rocha L, Beckman B: Soft Palate Advancement Flap for Palatal Oronasal Fistulae. J Vet Dent. 27(2):132-33, 2010.

[60] Niemiec BA: Pathology in the Pediatric Patient. in, Small Animal Dental Oral & Maxillofacial Disease (Niemiec BA (Ed)). Manson Publishing, London, pp. 89-126, 2010.

[61] Hale FA (2005). Juvenile veterinary dentistry. Vet Clin N Am, Sm Anim Pract 35:789–817, 2005.

## Appendix 1: Recommended equipment for extractions

There are a plethora of equipment options for veterinary extractions. This author's recommendations for a basic surgical pack are listed and pictured below. Each practice should have multiple packs, using a separate sterilized pack for each patient. The minimum supply of hand instruments should include:
- A selection of various sizes of elevators
- Periosteal elevator
- Small scissors
- Small-breed sized extraction forceps
- Brown-Adson forceps
- Small needle holders
- Scalpel handle.

These instruments are available in prepackaged kits from a few different companies.[d][e]

Elevators come in many types and sizes. Some veterinary dentists recommend winged elevators, but this author prefers luxating elevators. Utilizing luxating elevators can markedly decrease extraction time, especially with feline extractions. A variety of sizes is essential, with 2, 3, and 5-mm sizes recommended as a minimum supply. (Figure A1) Additionally, a 1-mm sized luxating elevator can be beneficial for feline extractions. Curved and straight options are available, and both types have inherent strengths.

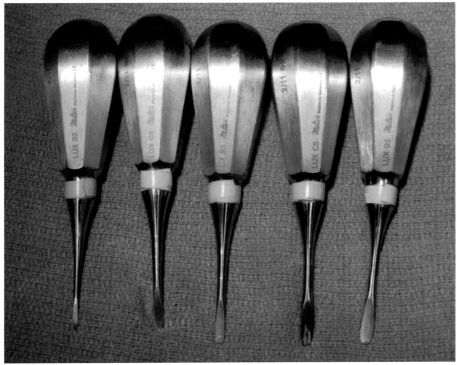

**Figure A1: Luxating elevators. C= Curved; S = Straight.**
**From left: 2-mm straight, 3-mm curved, 3-mm straight, 5-mm curved, 5-mm straight.**

[d] Niemiec Extraction Kit, Integra-Miltex, York PA
[e] Diplomate Extraction Kit: Dentalaire Products, Fountain Valley, CA

There are also numerous types of periosteal elevators, all of which are acceptable. This author prefers a Molt 2-4 and additionally a wax spatula. (Figure A2)

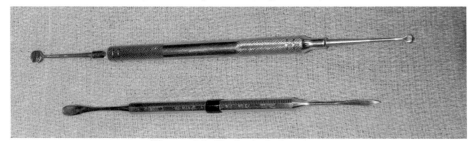

**Figure A2: Periosteal elevators.**
**Top: Molt 2-4**
**Bottom: Wax spatula 7A**

Use caution when selecting extraction forceps, as those designed for human dentistry do not work well in veterinary patients. More importantly, large sized forceps place too much force on the tooth adding risk of root/tooth fracture. Consequently, this author recommends only small breed sized extraction forceps. (Figure A 3)

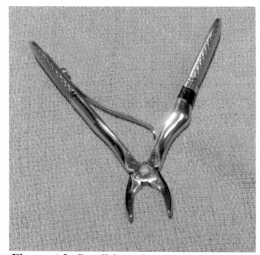

**Figure A3: Small-breed extraction forceps.**

Many varieties of surgical scissors are available. This author prefers a La Grange scissors.

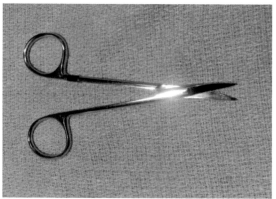

**Figure A4: La Grange scissors.**

The choice of forceps for use in dental/oral surgery is important, as 1x2 (rat tooth) forceps are too traumatic to the delicate gingiva. Brown-Adson (7x7) thumb forceps are recommended. Any type of needle holder can be used, but small sized instruments are preferred. Olsen-Hager and Castroviejo are typical choices. (Figure A5)

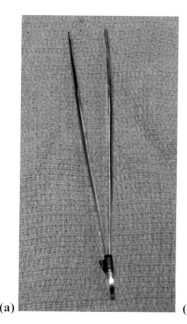
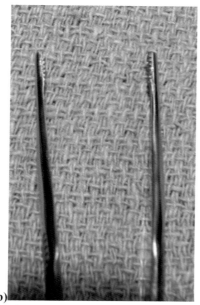
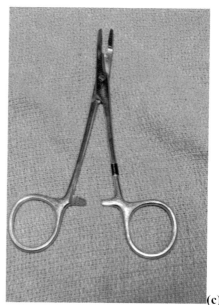

(a)    (b)    (c)

**Figure A5: Forceps and needle holders.**
a) **Brown-Adson tissue forceps.**
b) **Note the atraumatic "teeth" of the Brown-Adson forceps.**
c) **5 ½ inch Olsen-Hagar needle holders.**

The recommended instruments listed above are combined in a commercially available kit. This includes sharpening equipment and a sterilization cassette.[f]

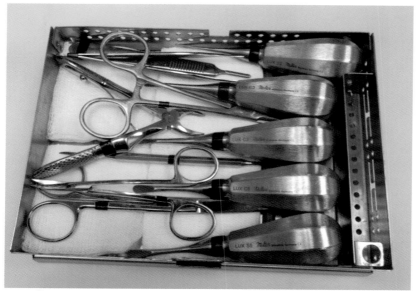

**Complete "Niemiec Extraction Kit" in a sterilization cassette.**

---

[f] Niemiec Extraction Kit: Intregra-Miltex, York, PA.

In addition to hand instruments, powered equipment is required for sectioning, buccal cortical bone removal, and bone smoothing/alveoloplasty. An air-driven high speed delivery unit is essential. It should be equipped with a high speed, low speed, and air-water syringe. (Figure A6)

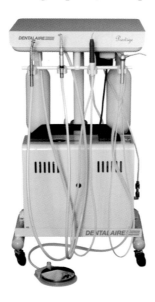

**Figure A 6: High-speed delivery unit**
**"Prestige": Dentalaire Products, Fountain Valley, CA**

Dental burs are available in various types and sizes. This author recommends carbide cross-cut taper fissure burs for sectioning and bone removal. These come in various sizes, with 699 being the smallest and 703 the largest. All sizes are useful. In addition, sizes 701 and 702 come in surgical lengths which provide increased surface area for cutting, and therefore speeds the sectioning/bone removal procedure. It is very important to note that dental burs are *disposable*. Moreover, they begin to dull after a very short period of time. Once burs dull (even a little), their cutting ability will decrease, which increases cutting time and subsequently increases thermal damage to the tooth and bone. Therefore, this author recommends a new bur for every patient. Coarse diamond burs are used for bone smoothing and alveoloplasty, and are available in flame or cylindrical options. Coarse diamond burs are disposable, but do last longer than carbide burs. (Figure A7)

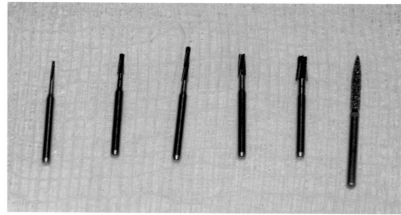

**Figure A7: Dental burs.**
**From left: 699, 701, 701 surgical length, 702, 703, flame shaped coarse diamond.**

64